1984

How

to Teach

Your Child

About Sex

BY Grace H. Ketterman, M.D.

Teenage Rebellion (with Truman E. Dollar)
How to Teach Your Child About Sex

How
to Teach
Your Child
About Sex

Grace H. Ketterman, M.D.

Fleming H. Revell Company
Old Tappan, New Jersey

Scripture quotations in this volume are from the King James Version of the Bible.

Library of Congress Cataloging in Publication Data

Ketterman, Grace H.
How to teach your child about sex.

Bibliography: p.
1. Sex instruction for children.   I. Title.
HQ53.K48   649'.65   81–1742
    ISBN 0–8007–1256–0   AACR2

Contents

Prologue

We live in the Western world, in a confusing climate of changing values, pleasure seeking, and permissiveness. While children are indulging in adult sexual activities at early ages, divorces are increasing. People who still care deeply about each other are getting divorced out of anger and social pressures. The children of divorce are tragically torn by their parents' battles. Venereal diseases are epidemic, and cures for them are becoming difficult to find due to resistance of the germs to medical treatment. The bitter battle of the sexes grinds on and the issue of gay rights has become a family issue as well as a political one.

With this grim picture of heartache, we can despair and predict disaster. Or we may seek the wisdom and courage to find our way out of the maze. In the library there is an index drawer half-full of cards describing how to make love, enjoy sex, be a man, be a woman, be nonsexist, teach a child about sex, and many more topics. The need for one more book may be questionable.

This book is an attempt to do something none of the others has done. Perhaps by seeing sex education as a circle, everyone can find a starting point and not feel defeated because of mistakes. Ideally, the development of healthy attitudes should take place in childhood. If it didn't happen that way in your experience, that's unfortunate, but it need not be devastating. You may learn such attitudes now. In learning and changing for the better, your children will have an example that carries over into every facet of life —not just in sexual areas.

Information about all sexual matters is important to you for your own happiness and the enrichment of your marriage. It is, of course, absolutely essential that your information is accurate if you are to teach your children about sex. Your ability to relate intimately and lovingly in your marriage will be increased and you will be able to carry over these lessons and teach your children the facts of life. Good information without good attitudes, however, is like teaching algebra without adequate knowledge about addition and subtraction.

No matter how healthy your attitudes or how complete your information, if you lack a sense of responsibility, you may end up doing nothing about teaching your child about sex. Being responsible in the totality of the way you live as well as in fulfilling your duties as parents sets the right example for your children.

The next part of the circle begins with your child at birth. Your attitude toward his tiny body sets the tone for his feeling about him or her self as a young person. How you handle the infant, enjoy him, and train him determines, to a large extent, the degree of confidence and even success he will attain. This success will include your child's idea of himself as a boy or girl and someday as a man or woman.

School-age children are the next arc on the circle, and they have special needs and feelings. They are struggling to give up the carefree time of early childhood. About the time that struggle is over, they have to give up their childhood completely to enter the even more frustrating period of adolescence. They need great understanding, acceptance, and wise discipline.

In adolescence, there is a convergence of child with adult in every aspect of life. The young person's life is characterized by confusion and extremes. Parents need to avoid riding this roller coaster with their child. They need to find and maintain some degree of calm in the center of their child's storm. As they do that, the child will gradually ride out the ups and downs and reach a reasonably successful adulthood.

Chapters on special issues that are part of our social and cultural environment complete this circle. The end of the circle is the beginning of the next one. And the hope of life lies in those who are willing to try to make their circle the best it can be so the next one can be even better.

Good sex education begins with your attitudes, depends on the accuracy of your information, and is learned only in an atmosphere of responsibility.

I hope this book will make your life as husband and wife a richer one, and your job as parents a more successful one. In breaking down life into its components, perhaps you will see more clearly how your job can be done. By understanding the physical aspects, emotional impact, intellectual influences, social interactions, and spiritual essentials, you may find, in a segment at a time, the ability to teach your child all about sex.

Part One

Parental Attitudes

1
Sexual Attitudes

Every parent teaches his or her child about sex, sometimes without even realizing it. Like it or not, it's a fact of life! A parent may do it in a well-planned fashion or haphazardly. Nevertheless, each child learns sexual lessons from his parents.

Many times I counsel people who have encountered serious problems that were related to their sexual experiences. Often I ask, "What did your parents teach you about sex as you were growing up?" Usually the answer is something like this one from a girl named Jenny: "My parents never did teach me about sex. They were too embarrassed about such things."

It was her parents' attitude that taught Jenny that sex was shameful and dirty, without their saying a word. As we examine Jenny's story more closely we will see how negative attitudes can be passed on from generation to generation.

Jenny's young uncle tried to force her, at the age of six, into sexual acts. She went to her parents, pleading for help. Her parents, refusing to accept any responsibility for such activities, said irritably, "You know our family would never do such things!" They ignored this sordid situation and Jenny was left defenseless through the rest of the vulnerable years of her childhood.

Out of these childhood experiences, Jenny emerged as a young woman with distorted sexual attitudes. She viewed sex as shameful and saw herself as ugly and unlovable. While she endured such negative feelings, Jenny also found herself to be easily aroused sexually. She was, in fact, preoccupied with such feelings and fantasies. The more she engaged in such thoughts, since she considered them so bad, the more ashamed she became. Jenny married a fine man who loved her a great deal. But it was almost impossible for her to believe in his love. Feeling as unworthy as she did, she became jealous and possessive of her husband. She feared that he would find someone better and more lovable than she was. Not knowing how to cope with Jenny's jealous accusations, her husband retaliated with anger, and a vicious circle developed.

As Jenny's children grew older, they witnessed repeated angry scenes between their parents, and became frightened and insecure. Growing up in such an environment, these children began to develop attitudes that were so like their mother's that their own future unhappiness seemed inevitable.

You can see from this example how negative attitudes are transmitted in the sexual aspect of life. Even beyond this, they permeate every area of life and are multiplied through each succeeding generation.

This vicious cycle can, however, be reversed. Through counseling and prayer, Jenny started to forgive and respect herself and her family. For the first time in her life, she began to see that she was a worthwhile person, worthy of being loved. Her husband and children, who really did love her, began to respect her, and she could finally accept their love.

Attitudes may be intentional or unconscious, and more often than not, they are communicated subtly. It is this very indirectness that makes attitudes so powerful and potentially dangerous that it is hard to argue or deal directly with them. A child, with his limited information and experience, is especially powerless to recognize or refute a negative attitude from a parent, so he usually grows up adopting such a position himself without realizing it or knowing where it came from.

Today's Western world focuses a great deal of attention on sex. Much of this exaggerates its importance and mistakenly implies that sex is the primary goal of living. In the first two chapters, we will examine healthy attitudes toward sex in five categories: physical, emotional, social, intellectual, and spiritual. At the conclusion of chapter two, we will discuss ways to change poor attitudes, how to acquire healthy ones, and how to pass these on to our children.

If, as you read on, you discover that you are uncertain as to just what your own attitudes are, or you realize that your attitudes are negative, be assured that you can change. That's what these chapters are about—understanding sexual attitudes and developing positive ones.

What is my physical attitude?

The human body is an amazing creation. So many billions of microscopic cells are similar and yet are different enough to make up all the systems of the body: skin and hair, muscles and tendons, bones, organs of sense, the respiratory system with which we breathe, the heart and circulatory system that supplies blood to all of our tissues, the excretory system that gets rid of the waste products of our metabolism, the digestive system by which we are nourished, the endocrine system by which we grow, mature, and age, and the reproductive system by which we reproduce ourselves in our children. That's quite a list! And with fairly minimal variations, you and every other human being have all these component parts.

Despite the amazing degree of perfection of our complex bodies, many people fail to appreciate and value themselves physically. Here's how to keep your attitude toward your physical self a positive one. List the characteristics about your body that you like. Use it to remind yourself that, as a little child once said, "God made me, and God don't make no junk!" If there are some things about your appearance you don't like, see if they can be changed. If, for example, you feel you are overweight, try a new diet or exercise routine. Learn to enhance the lovely parts of yourself rather than giving in to a sense of helplessness about your less desirable traits. You need not become egotistical, but it is important to be comfortable with your body and your appearance.

Next, take a look at your spouse. A bit too thin or fat, perhaps? But kind eyes, and a gentle face. Look for the beautiful aspects of that body and let yourself admire and love those aspects. Many a marriage is spoiled by critical attitudes. Rather than pointing out defects, try complimenting your spouse as you are learning to do to yourself. You may be amazed to find that your mate will begin to shape up without nagging from you!

Not only do you need to see yourself and your mate as physically lovely but you also need to know that in marriage, one of the finest experiences you were created to enjoy is the physical closeness that is called sexual intercourse. In order to realize this enjoyment, you need to feel free with one another as husband and wife. Showering together, dressing together, showing physical attention in creative ways such as tickling or touching one another at unexpected times, can be as important as sexual intercourse itself. In fact it is in the demonstration of simple affection that the groundwork is laid for a romantic sex life.

My daughter relates that the times in her childhood when she felt the most secure were related to her father's evening ritual. When he came home from work, he would go directly to the kitchen where I was preparing dinner. No matter what was cooking, it waited for the time it took for him to hold me in that moment of warm affection.

If you are instinctively a more reserved person, you may feel nervous at first about freely expressing yourself in a physical way. To become more comfortable, keep in mind your list of positive attributes and try showing your affection for your spouse in some new and creative way. This may be nonsexual because simply having fun with one another physically is related to children's play. Try to remember what sort of physical teasing you enjoyed as a child and experiment with a similar act as an adult. Once you and your spouse can laugh and play together outside the bedroom, it will become easier to take this happy attitude with you into the bedroom.

Within marriage, a husband and wife can physically enjoy one another without restrictions. Only a sense of respect and regard for the other's personal preference should limit the freedom you may enjoy. Your behavior and attitude toward each other will teach your children, more than words, about their own future marriages.

What is my emotional attitude?

Now we will explore an area of life that is more difficult to understand because it is less tangible than the physical aspect. The interaction of our sexual attitudes and our emotions is important, but it is both profound and complex.

Many careful studies have been done about infants and their inborn emotions. At birth, these studies reveal, babies have only two emotions: fear and anger. Fear is evidenced at a sudden jolt or a loud noise. Even at three weeks of age, my grandson responded to the noisy barking of our dog with a sudden loud cry and an expression of surprise and fear. At discomfort or frustration, anger is the clearly apparent emotion. An observing mother quickly recognizes the difference between these two responses. While newborn babies stimulate all sorts of love in their parents and grandparents, they do not show evidence of feeling love until they are somewhat older.

It is from our inborn anger that all of our aggressive feelings grow: irritation, frustration, rage, righteous indignation, and many other variations that you may name. From fear branch all the vulnerable emotions: worry, panic, inadequacy, shame, anxiety, and many more. When a child's early fears are relieved by love and protection, he will develop trust and learn to love and be loved. But when he is treated with anger or abuse and is taught to be overly aggressive, his ability to love will be lessened to some degree.

In no other part of life are emotions and physical functioning so obviously related as in sexual relationships. When the attitudes of both husband and wife are basically loving and trusting, their sexual experiences will be full of fun, tenderness, and sensitivity. In few parts of life is there such intertwining of giving and receiving, playfulness and intensity, and sharing of joy, as in healthy sexual intimacy.

Many people do not enjoy this ideal sex life because they have been taught to deny their emotions, both positive and negative, in all aspects of their lives. It is difficult for many people to even identify their own feelings, much less to share them with their spouses, because of childhood influences. The way adults respond to the expressed feelings of a little child sets the pattern for the way that child handles those emotions later on. It is as adults that we reap the harvest, good or bad, of this early implanting of attitudes. As adults, the way we express our emotions affects every aspect of our lives as we relate to others.

Emotions left unexpressed or misunderstood begin to create a barrier between two people. If allowed to continue, this barrier can become a wall. Such misunderstanding often is due to the fact that many people have more than one "layer" of feelings. On the surface they act one way while underneath they feel quite the opposite. Efforts to understand and care about the deeper feelings of the other person will create a bond of love and provide protection for the vulnerable feelings underneath.

My grandson, at two, dramatically demonstrated this fact. One day when I was baby-sitting with him, he abruptly left our playing and went to his bedroom. After a short time, I looked for him and found him staring moodily out of his window. At the sound of my voice, he yelled, "Grandma, go out of my house!" Since he usually was happy, I sensed that something lay under his angry outburst. After thinking for a minute, I replied, "Andy, you're sad that Mommy is gone, aren't you? If I weren't here, she would be with you. Right?" Instantly his anger dissolved into the sad tears he really felt, and he let me comfort him in my arms.

Had Andy not been able to share his vulnerable feelings with an understanding and caring adult, he would have felt safer to stay angry. Many adults have developed a habit of protecting such vulnerable feelings as hurts, disappointment, and loneliness with a facade of anger. You can see how such a habit on the part of one or both spouses can even interfere with their lovemaking.

It is difficult for many people even to identify their own feelings, much less share them with their spouses. Therefore, it is vitally important to look beneath the surface words and behavior of a child or a spouse to find the real feelings. This is listening with the heart as well as the ears.

To love someone is to trust him with your deepest feelings— even those you might not recognize without the help of the other person. Love is being sensitive to and protective of the tender feelings of another and is, therefore, a safe climate for the sharing of such emotions.

Questions About Feelings

Sometimes a protective wall may become so big that it not only protects those vulnerable feelings but it also buries them. It is possible to be so angry for so long that one may no longer recognize the vulnerable feelings below the wall of anger.

If this is true in your life, answering the following questions may restore your awareness of such feelings. Later, we will find ways to resolve these feelings.

How did your parents show the way they felt about each other? How did they look at one another? Were their actions thoughtful and kind? One of my favorite memories is of an every-Sunday-morning picture of my mother and dad. No matter how hurried we were (and with seven of us children, that was lots!) they always found time to stand and embrace in a secluded hallway. I would sit in my little rocking chair, quietly watching as my father's arms would hold Mom ever so tenderly as he kissed her soft cheek and then her neck. Their eyes were only for each other in that moment, and I doubt they ever knew the warmth and safety I felt in their commitment to love each other forever.

How do you feel about yourself? Are you worthy of being loved?

In the story of Jenny, her husband and children loved her very much. But for years, she could not accept their love because she had never learned to love herself. People who struggle with a sense of inadequacy or inferiority often have trouble becoming either emotionally or physically intimate.

How do you feel toward your spouse? Do you have a difficult time letting go of resentments?

If this is your problem, you may find the following technique helpful. Make a list of everything you resent about your spouse. A friend of mine had a list containing fifty-four items. Take time alone to think in an understanding way about why your spouse does each of the annoying things. By understanding, you will be ready to choose to truly forgive your spouse for every single offense. You need to do this, by the way, entirely within yourself in order to avoid arguments. Then every day, keep your mind and heart clear of resentments in the same way. On a day-to-day basis, you may discover areas that are so difficult to understand that you will need to discuss them with your spouse. Try to do this without making accusations or threats.

Is your own sexual gratification more important to you than that of your spouse? If one of you is in the mood for sex and the other is not, how do you resolve the conflict?

In a recent court case that received nationwide media coverage, a husband was put on trial for allegedly raping his wife. A friend, allying himself with the husband, said, "It's my wife's obligation to satisfy me whether she wants to or not." This comment reflects a selfish attitude and may result in the use of sex as a weapon in a power struggle.

Communication is the key to resolving this conflict. If each spouse expresses the real need and vulnerable feeling instead of angrily demanding his own gratification, the power struggle will be eliminated. Efforts to understand the needs of the other person, as well as one's own, and respond to these in a loving way, will create a bond of true intimacy.

Are your feelings easily hurt? How do you take care of these hurts? You may "lick your wounds" in martyrish silence; maybe you vow to get even; perhaps you cry and scream out the hurts in an argument. None of these methods is likely to heal hurt emotions.

Healing is possible by remembering that neither you nor your spouse is an ogre. Husbands and wives almost never plan to be cruel to each other. If one hurts the other, it is almost always, at least at first, by an accident, such as the misunderstanding of a word or a look. Sometimes one takes out on the other a problem from work. Rather than finding out why the spouse did the hurtful act, the victim is likely to retaliate in some fashion, and a pattern is started that may become a warfare of increasing cruelty. Checking out the real meaning of or the reason for an imagined attack, on the other hand, can keep alive an open and friendly communication, resulting in healing and a growing trust and love for each other.

How do you apportion your energy supply? Do you budget some energy for the expression of your feelings?

Each of us has a limited amount of time and energy. Sex, without deeply loving emotions, is not satisfying. Since such emotional expression requires energy, you need to save the time and energy for this part of your life.

The story of Marianne and Tom illustrates this point. Marianne had a demanding career, and by the end of her grueling days, she was not at all interested in sex. Tom was understanding, but often felt hurt by her insensitivity to his needs. Finally, Marianne quit work to raise their children. Having time and energy to spare, she found that she anticipated their sexual intimacy rather than dreading one more demand on her limited strength.

In order to keep alive the romance of marriage, sexual relations are important (although by no means is this the only or even the main ingredient!). To achieve a good sex life, you need to budget your time and energy, be sensitive to each other, be open and honest without self-pity or blame, and be creative in showing your love. This demands loving outside of the bedroom as well as in it, in all the little ways you can think of.

In a recent magazine article, I read about a wife and husband who put toothpaste on each other's brush if they woke up first. A tiny thing to do, but a loving way to wake up in the morning.

Contrast that with the story of my friend, whose husband could be thoughtless and rude. One day she asked, wistfully, "Honey, do you *really* love me?" Grabbing her hand, he replied, "Come with me to the bedroom, and I'll show you I do!" It was in the kitchen and the yard that she needed his love. The bedroom, tragically, proved nothing.

I hope from this list you may find the areas (if there are any) of

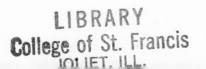

your emotional life that need some revamping. Please don't feel discouraged if you have discovered problems. Such a discovery is the vital first step toward a beautiful change for you and your spouse.

A change for the better in my marriage came about through the following painful experience. For many years, my husband would say to me on occasion, "Grace, you're such a martyr!" By "martyr" he meant that I was acting sad and hurt, when in reality my deeper feeling was anger. I knew, of course, that he was wrong! I had grown up in a family where I saw a relative who could act so hurt that I would often feel extremely guilty for hurting her, even though I never intended to do that. I had vowed and worked endlessly to avoid copying such problem behavior, so I knew I was not being a martyr. There came a day, fortunately, when I played that role so compellingly that even I had to admit it was true.

Early in our marriage, my husband made strict demands that I account to him for all the money I spent. He intended that to accurately keep our accounts, but I interpreted it as selfish and domineering. I tried to make him understand my need for a small amount of money that was strictly mine, to do with just as I pleased. He held firm: every dollar must be recorded. I finally burst into tears of despair. But even as I wept, I had to admit that I was really furious. He was unreasonable, and there were ways to keep accounts that could allow me some "mad money"! The argument itself was forgotten, however, as I finally recognized the way I covered my honest anger with tears. Those tears really were my soggy weapon!

Now I didn't admit that I was playing martyr right away! I struggled with my pride, my need to be right at all costs, and just giving in to the realization that my husband was right. I remember walking through the house, trying painfully to rationalize my way out. But at last I capitulated, went to my husband, and admitted this annoying trait. I vowed to change if he would help me, and change I did—slowly, and with many failures along the way. But no growth or change could have happened at all until I realized the problem.

2
More About Attitudes

While you are now discovering the positive attitudes toward your physical self and your spouse, and you are growing in healthy emotional attitudes, let us add the third task: understanding the intellectual component of positive sexual attitudes.

What is my intellectual attitude?

Your intellect is like a computer. It will, when operated correctly, take information, sort out the false from the true, test out the results, and store away experiences in a memory bank to be used as needed. Problems with this system arise when the information is faulty and when people fail to check it out. Information needs to be tried out to see whether or not it correlates with God's truth in the Bible and to find out if it works in the laboratory of human relationships. What we are discussing now are facts rather than feelings.

Difficulties in life as well as in marriage can be resolved intellectually by giving them careful consideration, evaluation, and analysis without allowing one's feelings to influence the outcome.

The following four steps are useful in solving such problems: 1. Be aware that the problem exists.   2. Make a conscious choice to resolve the problem.   3. Develop your willpower and self-discipline.   4. Remember that it takes hard work and tenacity to resolve most problems.

Awareness

By the time most people marry, they are old enough to have developed a series of behavioral and emotional patterns that are habits. They no longer think about them or are aware of them. Here is an example. When I was a child, I lived on a farm on the Kansas plains, where it could be extremely cold in the winter. Our house was not well heated and my feet would be cold as I brushed my teeth. I learned to stand on one foot, with the other foot balanced on top of it, so only one would get cold at a time! I thought I was very smart, but this became such a habit that many years later, in a warm house, and even in the hot summertime, I would stand like a bird on one foot to brush my teeth! Only after many years did my husband tell me that I looked silly doing that, and it annoyed him. He was right, and I could, with effort, change that habit—but only after I became aware of it and aware that it bothered my husband.

There are limitless differences between any two people coming from different families and having variations in beliefs, values, and expectations. Many times it is the expectations that may "do us in." Because my father always locked the doors at night, I entered marriage expecting my husband to make the house safe at night (and expecting him to be like my dad in other ways, as well). He wasn't, of course, like my father, and I began to fear that he really didn't love me since he was unwilling to lock the doors (to protect me). Many years passed, however, before I was clearly aware of feeling unloved. I just knew that bad, uneasy feelings were developing toward a good man. Once I was aware of these feelings and their cause, I could reprogram my computer with accurate information and come out with logical results. The true facts are that my husband, though unlike my father, is still a fine man. He came from a family where the doors didn't have to be locked. He did and does love me. And I can easily lock the doors, myself.

Awareness of feelings and facts demands that we be willing to stop expecting and begin exploring with our intellects.

Power to Choose

A dear friend of mine has had professional counseling over a period of years for various family and personal problems. He says that without a doubt, the most valuable of all the insights he has gained is the fact that he has the power of choice. His words are profound and as I have deeply explored this idea, I have become aware that of all God's creation, mankind alone has the power to choose intelligently. Animals may be trained or conditioned to choose, but as far as we know, they cannot intelligently do so.

It is relatively easy to see that one can choose how to act or even what to believe. Standing on two feet while brushing my teeth was not too hard. But I struggled endlessly with accepting the fact that I also have the power to choose how I will feel! Many people simply can't accept this fact at all. It is, nevertheless, true. I hate to remember the years when I would say (usually to someone I really cared about), "You make me so mad!" or "You hurt my feelings!" The truth is this: What that person did or said triggered an old reaction habit in me. Years ago, as a child who was quite helpless, some similar experience touched my vulnerable feelings, and I was unable to cope with that situation or work out its resolution. So I became angry to protect myself. As an adult, no longer helpless, I still really angered myself!

As adults, when we become aware of bad (painful) feelings, there are three simple steps we may choose to take to restore positive feelings. First, name the feeling, as accurately as possible. This is getting into an intellectual state rather than the helpless emotional state. Second, think about why the feeling has occurred. Avoid thinking in "you make me" terms and honestly look at yourself. Is the upset feeling coming from old habit patterns, or is the problem a here-and-now one? Whatever it is, define it clearly. Third, make a choice about dealing with the defined problem. The choice must be something one can constructively do alone, and not someplace the other person can go with it!

The most obvious of all personal choices, it seems to me, would be to choose to have good feelings and to encourage others to do the same. This is not only logical but scriptural as well. In many places in the Bible, we are told to avoid bitterness, wrath, anger, and evil of all sorts and cultivate the growth of love, joy, peace, gentleness, goodness, and so forth. I have known some people who seem to believe that enduring bad feelings is their burden to bear in life. Even if this is an unconscious belief, these people cannot be truly happy with themselves or with life. They can, however, learn to choose good feelings. I have developed a policy whereby I keep loving relationships active with everyone I know by resolving misunderstandings as they arise. You may choose your own life-style, but I recommend that you live lovingly!

More tensions and resentments come out of poor communication than from any desire to hurt or pull away from one another. These unresolved misunderstandings can spoil not only your sex life but your marriage and family relations as well. A major part of maintaining good attitudes demands clear communication, and that necessitates both awareness and choices. When you listen with your heart and eyes as well as your ears, you are communicating effectively. And if you will learn to ask and explain until what is said is close to that which is heard, you will be there.

Self-discipline

Now that you know you can choose how to think, act, and even feel, you need to discover the principle of using your will to make yourself do what is right and positive. I really wanted to cling to my belief that I was not a martyr and that my husband was wrong and mistaken about that. I had to swallow a huge gulp of pride in admitting that it was I who was wrong. It required awareness, a choice to be honest, and a large quantity of self-discipline to make myself admit to him that he had won our long-standing battle. But that's only how it seemed at the time. Actually I won, too, because I became a better person through that experience and our relationship grew as well.

If you grew up with inconsistent discipline from your parents, you will find self-discipline very hard. It is, however, by doing really difficult tasks that we learn the thrill of accomplishment and begin to enjoy being the person God intended us to be.

Work

According to a scientific definition, work is the process whereby energy is used to accomplish a given task. Actually, intellectual work is required to gain awareness, make choices, and exert self-discipline. It is also the factor that will see us through the process of growth and change that will produce those healthy inner attitudes. Work is closely connected with the will and discipline.

A relative of mine works part-time on a bridge-construction crew. On one occasion the men were asked to volunteer to go some distance for their next day's job. To the surprise of the older volunteers, a teenager, new to the group, volunteered to be ready to leave by four o'clock the next morning. In the early darkness the men met to drive together, and waited as long as they could for the young man, who never came. The following day, at a job closer to his home, he returned to work. One of the men asked him what had happened the previous day. His reply is classic: "Well, you see, I always wanted to see what it felt like to get up early in the morning, when it's still dark. I set my alarm and I got up. But I decided I didn't like it, so I went back to bed!" There are many people who "set their alarms" and their awareness is awakened. They even make the choice to get up and get dressed. But they fail to discipline themselves to follow through with the work! And, unless the job gets done, the first steps are useless.

A college friend of mine shared a practical philosophy of her uncle, who valued the willpower it takes to work effectively to the completion of a job. Every day this man would make himself do something he truly disliked, and he stopped himself, at least once a day, from doing something he wanted very much to do. Whatever your plan is to make yourself work at the changes you want, just complete the task. You're worth it!

In making changes of the type we are talking about, there are many discouragements. Habits are powerful, and we may automatically fall back into old ways, rather than forming new ones. In fact, we may doubt that the new habits will work at all. During such times, we each need a friend who is trustworthy and encouraging. Be sure, if you are committed to making a major change, to plan to work with such a person. Furthermore, it is important to expect a long, hard struggle. It took me several years to change some bad habits I had formed. But once the new pattern became automatic, I knew that it had been well worth the effort.

What is my social sexual attitude?

Now that you have achieved a positive physical image of yourself and your spouse, you express your emotions freely and naturally, and your intellectual attitudes are clear, you are ready for the consideration of sexual attitudes in social situations.

Some people see a threat in almost any social encounter. At the other extreme are those who attempt to dominate a social event. People who feel physically ugly, emotionally fearful or inadequate, and mentally confused, are ready prey for social blunders. The man who feels inferior often tries to cover this with a "macho" mask that actually fools others and even himself. Women may play the same game, usually using a mask of helplessness that gets all sorts of attention from the men who need to be "macho." On the other hand, insecure people may try the old "fade into the woodwork" act and be so socially withdrawn that they and people around them are miserable.

It is important that socially you see yourself as a fine and interesting person, with topics of interest to share and much to learn. Most people want someone to listen to them and show an interest in their affairs. To be the most appreciated person in nearly any group, ask people questions and respond to their conversation. Usually, you won't even get a chance to talk about yourself!

Not only does this type of social interaction help you to feel at ease and help others to feel important but it also eliminates the temptation to play risky sexual games. When you show genuine interest in others, and are honest with yourself, you can enjoy real relationships. You do not have to pretend anything and you will never find yourself in a corner with some explaining to do to your own spouse or someone else's!

Sometimes we think of social attitudes in life as existing only outside of the family. Many people (I used to be one of them!) act quite differently at home than in social situations away from home. You may find it enlightening to step back and compare the way you are at home and elsewhere. Is there a difference? Which way do you like best? Being real is making the way we feel, the way we look and act, and the way we talk all match. This should be the same at home as in any other situation.

One day I sat in my office with a young woman. She was weeping copiously, as she told me how badly her parents had treated her and that she just wished someone loved her. Being by nature and choice a loving person, I found myself, to my surprise, feeling angry instead of sympathetic with this girl. As I looked at her whole body I saw why. There was an angry set to her mouth and her fists were clenched. She was, as she admitted later, deliberately trying to make me feel sorry for her rather than help her face her need for honesty.

This kind of manipulation is common within families as well as in psychiatrists' offices and in business and social situations. Whether it is planned or unconscious, it takes away trust from relationships and replaces it with resentments and doubts.

Being honest and open, on the other hand, may also be harmful when that honesty is blunt or rude. I have seen families who were certainly accurate in their assessments of each other, but they were insulting and cruel in the way they communicated their criticisms. Even humor may be cruel in its expression. Teasing one another may become so intense that it seriously hurts the one being teased.

To develop an atmosphere at home that promotes both personal growth and interpersonal warmth and safety is a challenge. It requires the underpinnings of love, respect, and kindness. There was a time when I worked harder to please and understand friends than I did my own family. Their opinions seemed more important. That is no longer true, and I have learned to cherish the respect and love of my husband and children above all others. The social environment of our homes prepares our children for their social lives outside the home and is the model for their own homes later on.

What is my spiritual sexual attitude?

We humans are many-faceted creatures: physical, emotional, intellectual, and social. But we also are spiritual beings. If we omit any one of these qualities, we are incomplete.

Yet throughout the history of the Christian church, there have been individuals and groups who believed that to be close to God and truly spiritual was to deny one's sexuality. Biblical writings are remarkably candid about sexual matters. The stories of David, Saul, and all of the great heroes of the Bible reveal active sex lives. The only searing condemnation of sexual behavior is related to the dishonesty of adultery, the violence resulting from coveting another's spouse, and unnatural sex of incest and homosexuality. Jesus added to this list the deeper insight and level of honesty that is part of coveting. He said, "You have heard it said, in the olden days, 'Thou shalt not commit adultery.' But I tell you, whoever looks on a woman [for today we need to add, or a man] to lust after her has already committed adultery in his heart" (*see* Matthew 5:27, 28). Lust needs to be defined as simple physical desire without love or commitment. Man was created for a higher way of life than were the animals.

In the story of the Creation, God saw that it was unfair for Adam to live alone and in the most beautiful way, God created woman from Adam's own flesh to be his companion. Only later were they told to bear children. Read it for yourself in Genesis.

One of the love classics in the world's literature is the Song of Solomon. It has been called a metaphor of God's love for His followers. But it is written in beautifully descriptive human terms. In fact, when God was looking for the best description of the relationship of His Son, Jesus Christ, with those who believe in Him, He grouped all of them together and called them His Bride. The very highest and holiest relationship between God and man, then, is like the ultimate intimacy of the honeymoon of the bride and groom. I know of no higher permission for or blessing on the sexual expression of love between a husband and wife than God's Word puts forth.

So much for this lengthy discussion of good sexual attitudes. Just how, simply and specifically, can you acquire such attitudes? Some of you are the unwilling victims of old "tapes" that keep telling you sex is ugly and embarrassing. Many of you are confused and don't know where you stand on sexual attitudes. This section will help you to understand and clarify your position.

Helpful Rules for Healthy Attitudes

Many of our problems with poor sexual attitudes were either taught or modeled by our parents. I want to be careful in saying this, because psychiatrists have a reputation for blaming their patients' faults on their parents. This is not at all what we intend. Your parents, as you do, did the best they could in raising their children. But they, like you and I, made mistakes. Some of what they taught you was inaccurate information, and it won't work in your computer any better than it did for them.

Here are some basic rules that may make it easier for you to find and adopt good sexual attitudes in all areas of your life.

Rule 1. Think about all of your present attitudes and beliefs about sex. Are they positive and wholesome, or do you find areas of embarrassment? Do you men feel that you are superior to women? Or secretly, do you women believe that you are really the better sex?

Sort through your beliefs and prejudices, and choose the attitudes that are kind and positive. You may find it helpful to discuss these ideas with your spouse or a trusted friend. Reading may be useful. Whatever it takes, get your ideas clear.

Rule 2. Talk about your new or reaffirmed beliefs and ideas until they really become yours. Practice the healthy attitudes until they become automatic.

Following this rule should result in your becoming just as comfortable discussing sexual issues as any other issue. You may find that you no longer consider dirty jokes funny (even secretly!). You may not be as shy and you probably won't be flirtatious around the opposite sex.

Rule 3. Stay free from the damaging results of persistent anger and fear. These two emotions, you may remember, are present at birth. They may be lifesaving when they are recognized and used properly. But they become emotionally crippling when they control us. Many times these feelings have been buried so deeply within us that we are hardly aware of their existence.

As you learn to face yourself more honestly and comfortably, however, you may become aware that anger and fear are defeating your work toward developing good attitudes. If you cannot understand and overcome these negative forces by yourself, do consult a good counselor. There are many fine people who are trained to help you work out such problems.

Rule 4. Feel good about yourself! You may not even realize that you have negative attitudes toward yourself. And please don't make up such attitudes if they aren't there! I find, however, that a great many people do have self-doubts or feel downright awful about themselves. Such feelings grow out of experiences early in life in which we failed or were excessively criticized.

An eighth-grade girl was sent to me for an evaluation because she was failing in school, refused to take part in school activities, and was isolating herself from friends. As we talked, I saw a family pattern of excessive criticism, bickering, and anger. I asked her if anyone at all was proud of her for something. Wistfully she thought and tears welled up in her sad, brown eyes as she whispered, "Just my dog!" I was grateful that day for the pets that give such children some sense of love and importance. But I was reminded of the many people, both adults and children, who have never known that glow of pride when someone says, "Hey! That's good! You're going to make it!"

If you are one of those people who never had a chance to be a "star," you can become one now. A star is someone who stands out in the crowd, and I have an idea that in one degree of brightness or another, God would want each of us to shine in the crowd.

This time, you be the judge as well as the performer. Improve your skills at work, at home, in a hobby, or as a good neighbor until those skills are the very best you can make them, and then make them a little bit better—because most of us can do better than we think we can! And then feel good about what you've done. It's all right to ask your spouse or a good friend for their approval of your efforts. As you find your abilities growing, you will feel better about yourself, and all of your attitudes in life will become more positive. Your sexual attitudes are sure to be included!

Rule 5. Feel loving toward others. As we learn to really love ourselves, it becomes easier to accept and love the others in our lives. As we think about teaching children about life and specifically about sex, it becomes clear that they will learn best when they are secure in the love of their parents.

Rule 6. Explore God's love. One really exciting fact about the life of Jesus was His acceptance of all sorts of people just as they were. The lepers, the adulterers, the publicans and sinners were loved by Him and healed by Him. When our own love runs out, His supply is endlessly available to replenish us.

Teaching Healthy Attitudes

Having acquired sexually positive attitudes and feelings for oneself is one thing. How to teach these to children is quite another. There is much, however, of such teaching that is easy because children are so sensitive. Young children will watch parents and tend to absorb their attitudes. But here also are some guidelines that may help you more specifically:

Accept your child and love him exactly as he is. If your attitudes favor boys over girls (or vice versa) it will hurt your daughter and may give your son a superiority complex that may hurt him, too. It is tempting to cling to a dream you've always had of a certain kind of child—a great basketball player or a champion swimmer. As your child grows, it may be that he will exceed your dreams. But it often happens that he is too short for basketball or is afraid of water. Can you turn off your dream and sincerely love and approve of your child as he is? If your attitude toward him is one of disappointment, he will sense it. Furthermore, he will believe that he, not you, has failed and may give up or perhaps retaliate by hurting you in some way. I've worked with hundreds of rebellious young people. I have rarely seen one who was not emotionally hurt by his own parents. Unconditional acceptance is a prime factor in self-esteem, and that is essential to the future well-being of your child.

Train your child well. Decide how you want him to behave and then by your example and good discipline teach him how to measure up to those standards. Be careful to ask of your child only what he is capable of doing. Expecting the impossible is defeating. Expecting too little is humiliating. As you practice this sort of discipline in the broad scope of your child's life, you will unknowingly be strengthening him in sexual areas as well.

Set a good example by treating each other well as husband and wife.

My daughter used to be horrified at the way one of her friends would treat her mother. One day after visiting in their home, she said, "Mother, I know now why Gayle treats her mom the way she does. While I was at her house, her dad came home. You should see the way he treats her mom!" Sexual attitudes in that family were marred by the father's attitude of disrespect for the mother.

Be as careful to praise your child as you are to criticize him. It's easy to focus on the negatives, as parents, because it is our duty to help a child overcome the weaknesses he shows. We may fail to understand that the strength and courage by which he can overcome, are born of his successes. As a child learns to succeed at stacking blocks, learning to spell, throwing a ball, and getting along with friends, he will learn to succeed as a spouse and parent.

Be as consistent as you can. When you give praise one day for a clean room and fail to notice it the next, a young child may not know whether cleaning his room is important. If you scold or punish him for tracking mud on the rug on Tuesday, but on Thursday mud tracking is ignored, again he will be confused.

Being a parent is not easy. It must go on whether or not you are tired and even when things at work are a mess, or you and your spouse have had an argument. Once you give in to the reality of the difficulties and find the superhuman strength just to "do it," it becomes possible. And if you hang in there long enough, the rewards of seeing your children become warm, loving adults will convince you that it truly was worth all it took.

3

Information

Before you can teach your children about sex or answer their questions, you need to be sure you know the facts yourself. Definitions of many common sexual terms are, therefore, included in this chapter to help you clarify these facts.

The following story exemplifies the importance of having your facts straight for your own sake as well as that of your children.

A young couple came to me for help because the wife simply could not reach a sexual orgasm, or climax. She and her husband loved each other very much and both had tried everything they knew that might help her find real sexual fulfillment. After several years of searching, they came to me, hoping a psychiatrist could find the answer.

For weeks, we worked together checking out their beliefs about sex, their feelings toward each other, and their feelings toward themselves. There were a number of very real resentments and problems of a serious type from their childhood days. But even when these were resolved, Sherrie was as unsuccessful as ever in reaching that coveted experience.

One day, on a happy impulse, I asked Sherrie to describe to me exactly what she did experience, physically, at the end of their sexual relations. To my surprise and delight, she described a perfectly normal female orgasm. The erotic feelings would build gradually to an intensity that was broken by the soft muscular contractions of the climax, followed by relaxation and a peaceful warmth that was satisfying to her.

I was delighted to tell Sherrie that what she had just described was entirely normal and watched as the anxiety left her face and her body relaxed. She told me that she and her husband believed that this experience should be so intense that her whole body would quiver and the bed shake. Wrong information had partly spoiled their sex life for too long! Adequate information on the topic of sexuality is crucial. If your information is wrong or is inadequate, you may be in trouble.

The most important piece of information I want you to know is this: Sexual intercourse is a normal, natural, God-given part of life. Once you understand all that means, other sexual information will fall into place with balance and perfection. Sex is not, as some believe and our society advertises, the ultimate goal of life, an idol to worship, or a dream to pursue. It is as important as the ingestion of food, the respiration of air, and all the other processes of the body.

In fact, there is a level of sexual functioning that is nothing more than biological. Let's talk about the *physical* aspects of sex. As human beings reach sexual maturity (called puberty), their bodies begin to experience a new set of feelings. To be sure, even little children have pleasant sexual feelings when their genital areas are touched, but this is not of the same quality or intensity as adult sexual sensations. In almost every person, certain anatomical locations, when touched or even thought about, will give rise to sexual feelings or desire. These are called the erogenous zones (not to be confused with your erroneous zones!). The usual erogenous zones include the lips and mouth; the breasts, especially the nipples, the inner areas of the upper thigh, the labia, vagina, and clitoris in women; the penis and scrotum in men. Other parts of the body may come to be sexually stimulating, depending on conditioning and the association of these areas with sexual experiences.

Physical Attraction

It is ideal that sexual intimacy should be the ultimate physical expression of emotional love and respect and may even have spiritual implications. In actuality, however, it may fall far short of this lofty goal. Sexual relations may be nothing more than an expression of simple erotic arousal. Depending upon early-childhood experiences, energy levels, physical and mental sensitivities to sexual innuendos, and many other variable factors, some people are quickly and intensely sexually aroused and others much less so and more slowly.

It is at this point that your attitudes go into effect. If your attitude is one of self-gratification, you may give in to, or seek, sexual experiences wherever and whenever you choose. This seems selfish and exploitive. Such a choice, if it becomes a way of life, will limit the development of your whole being and will almost inevitably end up in frustration and disappointment for both you and your spouse.

Being physically attracted to a person other than one's spouse is normal, since sexual attraction is a biological function. This physical appeal implies nothing more and need not be acted upon.

I would like to discuss three concepts that emphasize how important it is to understand this kind of attraction.

1. If you find yourself in a situation that involves sexual feelings for someone other than your spouse, you need to know how to deal with it safely. Each individual needs to know himself and his areas of physical vulnerability so well that he can remain in control of himself in any situation.

An acquaintance of mine brags about his sexual exploits. One of his favorite stories is of attending a party where he met an attractive woman. Before the party ended, he had managed to seduce her in an upstairs bedroom. She later shared with a friend, "It was over before I knew what was happening." It is obvious that the woman failed to understand her areas of physical vulnerability. The dangers of sexual promiscuity are several: physical, emotional, and spiritual. Each of us needs to be aware of how and when we may become erotically aroused if we are to avoid such a dangerous way of living. We need to choose to control those sexual feelings and to avoid situations that involve temptation and opportunities to give in to such feelings.

2. If at some point in your life you have given in to the temptation of such a transient physical attraction, how have you dealt

with it? The most common reaction I have seen is to feel guilty. Guilt nearly always prompts a confession to someone—a friend, or even more often, the spouse. Such a confession, instead of helping, may cause more hurt and misunderstanding. Guilt is a positive force if it is understood and resolved. First, it can stop the destructive behavior because it is so uncomfortable. Second, guilt over such an episode can motivate self-understanding and self-discipline. But staying guilt ridden is unbearable, and should not happen. The resolution of guilt requires forgiving oneself and accepting God's forgiveness. Telling a spouse of such an experience usually causes immense pain and horrible misunderstanding and is not automatically necessary. Keeping such an experience between you and God may be the best course to pursue. What is critical and essential is for you to know God's restoration and forgiveness.

3. A husband or wife needs to understand that an episode of unfaithfulness by one does not necessarily mean a loss of love for the other. It doesn't even mean that one spouse wants an ongoing affair with someone else. It often means, simply, that the vulnerable one, due to a failure to control his or her physical urges, fell into temptation. In such a situation, an understanding and forgiving spirit, and a plan for avoiding repetition, can restore a good marriage.

A businessman recently called me about one of his employees. She had become emotionally upset at the discovery that her husband was seeing another woman. The employer said that he knew she would, of course, get a divorce, but he was concerned that she find help for her problems.

In talking with the woman, I learned that neither she nor her husband wanted a divorce. He was willing to give up the other woman and they were able to forgive and rediscover their love for each other. It is not necessarily a point of honor to punish the erring spouse by getting a divorce. At the other extreme, the concept of "open marriage" has been so widely advocated that to many people it is permissible to indulge in sexual relationships whenever and with whomever they please. Both of these philosophies represent a sad and dangerous commentary on today's culture.

You can choose to control your sexual urges, since you are so much more than a biological creature.

Within a good marriage, the enrichment of a mutually enjoyable sexual relationship can be increased by knowing each other's and one's own unique erogenous zones. The joy of giving and receiving physical pleasure is both an expression and a bond of married love. Despite a great increase in information about sex, many people still do not know that the wife, as well as the husband, may experience the joy of sexual fulfillment. A wise and loving husband will take time to help his wife become sexually aroused and brought to the sexual climax, called an orgasm. The wife, by understanding her body and the way God has created it, may freely respond to enjoy her own sexual experience.

Definitions

Now we will define some basic sexual terms. You need to know these facts if you are to teach your children correctly. We will first define a number of terms, then have a short discussion about anatomy and physiology.

Sex and Sexual Terms

Sex: This word simply means male or female. The sex of a baby tells us whether it is a boy or a girl. The word *sex* has also come to mean the act of sexual intercourse.

Sexuality: This word may also mean male or female, but accurately it includes all of the qualities or attributes of each sex.

Sexual intercourse: The most intimate of physical closeness in which the husband and wife are physically joined together. The husband's erect penis is inserted in the wife's vagina where, with rocking and thrusting movements, both reach a peak of sexual feeling called an orgasm. It results in the discharge of sperm in seminal fluid from the husband, and a wavelike contraction of muscles in the clitoris and vagina of the wife. It is usually highly pleasurable and unless preventive measures are taken, it may result in pregnancy. There are other means of sexual intercourse that have come to be acceptable in today's world,

Female Sex Organs

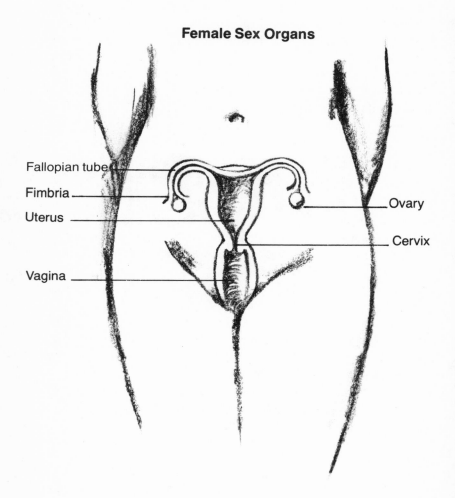

but they will not be included here.

Coitus; copulation: These are technical terms for sexual intercourse.

Foreplay: A term describing the early part of sexual intercourse. Most husbands and wives enjoy a period of affection with caressing, kissing, and simply enjoying the feel of their own and their spouse's bodies. This prepares them for coitus and makes their reaching the pleasure of a sexual climax more likely.

Sexual orgasm or climax: As described above, it is the peak of the sexual experience and is followed by a sense of great peace and relaxation. When the climax is not reached, it may leave one or both frustrated and uncomfortable.

Female Anatomy

Ovum: This is the female sex cell. It rests in a girl's ovary from birth, but at puberty it grows along with thousands of others. Once a month (sometimes twice) one ovum bursts out of its tiny pocket, is gently pulled up into one of the Fallopian tubes, and passes into the womb to be fertilized or discharged.

Ovary: Female sexual organ that is about the size of a small plum. It lies in the lower abdomen protected by the pelvic bone. Above it is the end of the Fallopian tube, called the "fimbria," which draws the ovum into the womb.

Tubes or Fallopian tubes: Literally hollow tubes connecting the womb with the ovaries. The end of the tube near the ovaries flares into an umbrellalike opening that, by its waving motion, draws the ovum into the tube. Gentle movement of the tube moves the egg on into the womb.

Uterus (womb): The place prepared to protect and nurture a developing fetus until it is a baby ready to be born. It is about the size and shape of an inverted pear. From each upper side extends the tube (Fallopian tube) that ends in the fimbria that rests over the ovary. The lower end of the uterus becomes the *cervix,* which is the opening through which the semen, loaded with sperm cells, enters during intercourse. The cervix contains many glands. They constantly put out small amounts of a whitish substance called mucus.

As the mucus slowly flows out through the vagina, it keeps this area clean and washes out bacteria.

Vagina: A tubular structure with soft walls leading from outside the body to the cervix. It directs the husband's penis to the proper opening to make conception possible, and it is the canal through which the baby passes at birth.

Urethra (female): The short tube leading from the urinary bladder to the outside of the body. It serves only as the passageway through which urine is voided, and has no sexual function.

Labia: Folds of skin, glands, and muscle fibers that fall together like lips, protecting the vagina from dirt or germs that could cause an infection. They are spread apart during intercourse to allow entrance of the penis.

Clitoris: A small (one-half inch or less) projection of tissue that is firm and contains many blood vessels. With the stimulus of sexual play or intercourse, it becomes erect and with the friction reaches a point of involuntary muscular contraction that extends to the vagina. It is extremely pleasurable, as is an ejaculation in the husband, and is followed by deep relaxation and a sense of emotional warmth. It is located in the midline of the body, just beneath the lower edge of the pubic bone.

Female Physiology

Menarche: The beginning of a girl's menstrual cycle. It first occurs about one year after the appearance of body hair under the arms and in the pubic area (groin).

Menstruation: The discharging of tissue, blood, and fluid from the womb when conception has not taken place. It occurs about once a month, lasts from three to seven days, and is often accompanied by some degree of discomfort.

Menopause: The time in midlife when a woman's hormone secretions decrease, causing her menstrual cycle to stop. About this time, ovulation stops and pregnancy is no longer possible. The age at which this takes place varies a great deal from the early forties to the early fifties.

Estrogen: The primary female sex hormone that is responsible, along

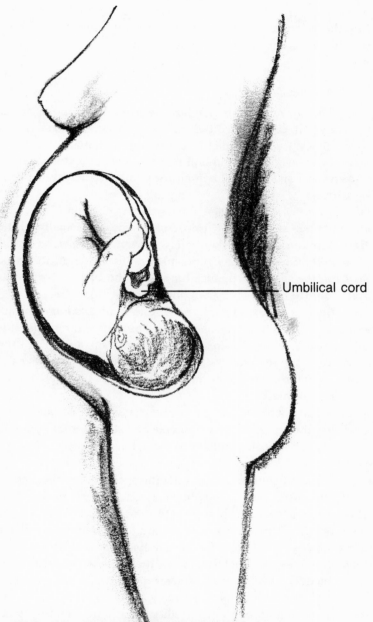

Umbilical cord

Baby Near Time For Delivery (9 Months)

with other hormones, for breast development, roundness of hips, and other feminine characteristics.

Male Anatomy

Sperm: The male sex cell. It is about the size of a pin point and is very active. It contains half of the material, called genes and chromosomes, that is needed to create a new human life.

Scrotum: A strong sac of skin and muscle fibers that is suspended between the man's legs and behind the penis. Inside rest the testicles or testes.

Testicles: Olive-sized male sex glands that make sperm cells and certain hormones, especially testosterone. They are usually a little different in size and one may be lower than the other.

Vas deferens: Similar to the Fallopian tube in a woman, this tube goes from the testes to the urethra inside the body. Sperm cells travel from the testicles to the penis through this tube.

Urethra (male): A tube leading from the urinary bladder through the penis and ending as an opening at the end of the penis. It is a highly useful structure since it also receives openings from the vas deferens, the seminal vesicles, and the prostate, as well as the bladder. A unique valvular arrangement prevents the flow of urine during sexual intercourse.

Seminal vesicles: Two small sacs near the urinary bladder and prostate within the pelvis. They help make and store seminal fluid, in which the sperm are suspended and carried in the process of ejaculation.

Semen: The thick substance in which the sperm are suspended. It is perfectly clean, but it does have an odor which some wives dislike. There is no need, however, to use chemicals to deodorize after intercourse, because in a few hours, most of it will have drained out and the body will cleanse itself internally.

Prostate gland: A gland that surrounds the urethra just below the urinary bladder. It helps make semen.

Penis: A male sex organ that is normally about five to seven inches in length and one to one-and-a-half inches in diameter. It is at-

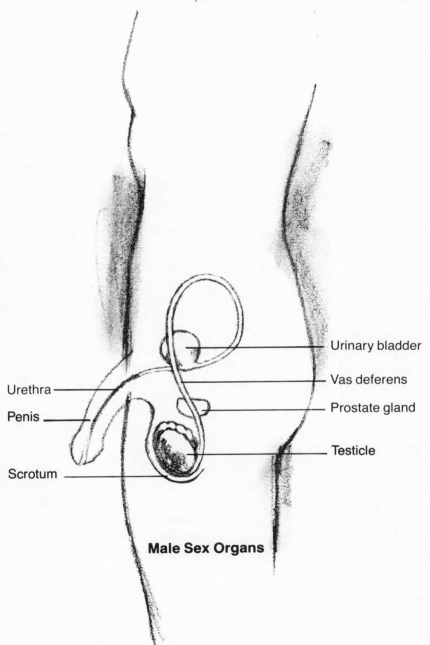

Male Sex Organs

tached to the body by muscles and skin and hangs between the legs and in front of the scrotum. Through it passes the urethra. Besides this tube, muscle fibers, and a thick protection of skin, the penis contains a rich network of blood vessels. When sexually aroused, these become distended with blood, causing the penis to become larger, firm, and erect.

Male Physiology:

Erection: The condition in which the penis automatically leaves its hanging position to protrude almost at right angle to the body. It is then ready for sexual intercourse and may be inserted into the wife's vagina.

Ejaculation: The discharge of semen from the husband's penis.

Premature ejaculation: The rapid reaching of the stage of ejaculation by the husband before the wife is ready for her climax.

Emission: Another term for ejaculation.

Nocturnal emission: Another term for a wet dream, this is the automatic discharge of excess seminal fluid and sperm during sleep. It is one of nature's ways of releasing sexual tension in a male.

Testosterone: The predominantly male hormone that produces the growth of body hair, the lower male voice, the growth and development of sperm in the testes, and the growth of the penis and of the body as a whole.

General

Hormones: Chemicals that are manufactured by a group of glands called the endocrine system. Masterminded by the hypothalamus and pituitary glands, this group includes the thyroid and parathyroid glands in the neck, the adrenal glands atop the kidneys in the small of the back, the ovaries and testicles. There is an amazingly intricate interaction of each of these on the others that keeps us functioning.

Chromosomes: A complex protein substance that carries the genes in a sex cell (sperm or ovum).

X and Y chromosomes: These very special chromosomes determine the sex of the fetus. The male sex cell has both X and Y chromosomes, while the female has two X chromosomes. Immediately prior to conception, a cellular division takes place in both the male and female sex cells, leaving either an X or Y half (male) or two X halves (female). The sex of the child depends on which male half-cell unites with the female half-cell.

Genes: Complex substances that are responsible for an individual's uniqueness: the color of the eyes and hair, shape of the nose and ears, fingerprints, and so forth. While certain family traits are handed on to new babies, each person is significantly different from every other due to the differences in genes.

Conception: The beginning of a new life by the actual union of a sperm with an ovum. Only one of millions of the active little sperm will reach the ovum. As soon as they have become attached by the mysterious magnetism that puts and holds these half-cells together, a protective shield is formed. No more sperm can enter, and they are all discharged back through the cervix.

Douche: This is the process by which some women choose to cleanse out their vaginas with disinfectants or water. At one time, doctors recommended this as a means of preventing conception and for internal hygiene or cleanliness. We know now that unless there is an infection, our bodies tend to cleanse themselves, as I have explained above. Be very careful, if you do use a douche, to use only a substance that your doctor knows is safe.

Contraception: This is the process of the prevention of conception, described above. There are many methods for this that are perfectly safe, will allow you to enjoy your sex life as husband and wife, and enable you to space and plan your children according to your needs and wishes. There is a complete discussion of contraception in chapter eleven.

Abortion: The loss of a fetus during the first three months of pregnancy. An abortion may occur spontaneously or it may be done deliberately by a doctor, if the mother chooses. While the latter is legal, it involves many moral issues that need to be considered. A spontaneous abortion may result from a defective fetus, a fall, an illness, or some abnormality of the mother's hormones or reproductive organs. A mother needs a doctor's care in such a situation.

Reproductive tract: In a woman, this includes the labia, the clitoris, the vagina, the cervix, the uterus, the tubes and fimbria, and the ovaries. In a man, the reproductive tract includes the scrotum and testicles, vas deferens, seminal vesicles, prostate gland, penis, and urethra.

Masturbation: The process of handling and manipulating one's own genitals to the point of a sexual orgasm, though the term is also used to describe stroking or stimulating one's body short of an orgasm.

Homosexual: One who is sexually aroused only—or primarily—by a person of the same sex.

Lesbian: A woman homosexual.

Bisexual: One who can become sexually involved with either sex.

Frigidity: The inability of a wife to enjoy a sexual orgasm. It falsely implies that she is emotionally "cold," and that is far from true in most cases.

Impotence: The inability of a husband to achieve either an erection or an ejaculation, or both. Most impotence and frigidity can be helped either medically or through counseling.

Pregnancy: The condition involving the nurture and growth of a fertilized ovum within the mother's uterus, to the time of birth. Except for the early loss of the fetus through abortion or miscarriage, this process takes about 280 days from the day of conception —about nine calendar months. When the baby's maturation process is just right, the mother's womb somehow knows that it must push the baby out. This process is called labor.

Umbilical cord: A connecting structure that carries nourishment from the placenta to the fetus during pregnancy.

Labor: The regular, firm contraction of the muscular walls of the uterus which slowly pushes the tiny baby (usually headfirst) through the cervix, down the vagina, and out into the world. This lasts from a few hours to nearly a day (an average of twelve hours for a first baby and five or six hours for later ones). Usually doctors give the mother a general or local anesthetic to make her comfortable during this process.

Natural childbirth: Many mothers want to feel all the processes of their baby's birth and be awake to see the new child. These mothers may ask their doctors to use little or no anesthetic. A recent trend to include fathers in the birth process is extremely fortunate, in my opinion. By a course outlined in the Lamaze method, husbands and wives attend classes during the pregnancy and the husband serves as his wife's "coach" during labor, helping her breathe and relax properly. He generally supports her through a difficult and sometimes frightening experience. The closeness this allows and the actualizing of becoming a father and mother together is exciting!

Caesarean section: This is a surgical procedure that is used when it may be unsafe or impossible for a mother to vaginally deliver her baby. A doctor will advise this carefully and only when he believes it to be necessary.

Miscarriage: The spontaneous birth of a baby between the third and sixth month of a pregnancy. It may be due to several causes: illness, accident, a slightly deformed or damaged cervix, an abnormal baby, and others. Usually this requires hospitalization for a short time to prevent complications and help the mother get her strength back.

Fetus: A medical term given to an unborn child. By the third month, however, this fetus looks like a tiny baby with fingers, toes, and all the parts of its body in evidence.

Premature baby: A baby born between the sixth and ninth months. Usually a six-month baby is too poorly developed to live outside the mother's body. But with great care and today's new techniques, its chances are considerably improved. By the seventh and eighth month, most babies can live, but they require very special care. An entirely new medical specialty called "neonatology" has been developed just to give tiny newborn babies a better chance to live.

4
More Information

I hope you found the last chapter helpful in clarifying some facts about sex.

Now let's discuss the emotional aspects of sex. We have already discovered in chapters one and two how fear, worry, anger, guilt, and resentment (to name only a few negative feelings) can completely block out your loving sexual feelings and desires.

We also described some ways to get rid of such feelings. So just let this be a reminder that if you want a fulfilling sex life as husband and wife, practice the understanding of each other that will allow you to forgive one another and stay warm and loving. As you love in your hearts, you will be able to express this in your physical relations.

Destructive Games

One of the major deterrents to this ideal understanding of each other is the unconscious playing of games. "Games" are a type of communication between two people. They are played unconsciously to satisfy the need for emotional attention. Unfortunately, they end in negative feelings on the part of one or both players. Clarifying the most destructive of these games may enable you to avoid or stop playing them.

Power struggle is the competition between two people for the dominant authority position. Someone has perceptively said that there are two battlegrounds on which most couples fight out their power struggles: One is money and the other is sex. We are concerned here only with the sexual aspect of power struggles.

When one partner is unsure of his importance as a person (and, therefore, is unsure of his importance to his spouse), he may unconsciously begin this game. Because of his negative self-attitude, he tries to compensate by convincing himself that he is able to control at least this one aspect of his life. He exercises this control by demanding or withholding sex at the expense of the other's desire. Now imagine what would happen if both partners played this game. These people would be fighting over sex or no sex when they really needed to know, "Am I an important person?" and "Do you really respect me and love me?"

The resolution and avoidance of this game depends on respecting and loving yourself, as we have discussed previously. You must define what you need and communicate this clearly. To admit your needs may require eliminating a false sense of pride. When you are clear about the cause of this game, it will be over and you will both win!

Jealousy is resentment toward anything or anyone seen as a rival for the attention or affection of one's spouse. This gamelike power struggle emanates from an unconscious sense of inadequacy. The jealous partner can never realistically get all the attention he demands. Any rival for the spouse's attention comes to be feared as more important or more lovable in the eyes of the spouse.

For a number of years in our marriage, my husband needed time and space to be alone. That was a brand-new idea to me because my parents were (and seemed to want to be) always together. I love my husband and felt I could never have enough time with him. So for years, when he would go away or sit in his study, alone, I felt abandoned and rejected. I suspected he had found another woman who was prettier or more desirable than I. My pride, of course, would not let me tell him how ugly and unworthy I often felt. And I suspect his pride wouldn't let him admit that all the responsibilities of a wife and family seemed heavy to him.

Had he told me about the stress he endured, and explained his needs clearly, or had I been better able to clarify my worries, we would both have avoided an element of misunderstanding over a number of years. In one of the ironies of life, when I finally understood and stopped feeling threatened by his needs, my husband no longer had the craving for so much space and time of his own!

This game is over when you know that you are the best person you can be and you no longer have to try to be perfect. Furthermore, the value of yourself comes from within you and not from the opinion of anyone else. Most important, knowing that you are created in the very image of God makes you priceless in His eyes!

Vengeance is getting even for hurts that have been inflicted by the partner. This game can involve the accumulation of slights, real or imagined, from many years, or only from a recent episode. The rule of this game is "Don't get mad. Get even." Getting even sexually may involve extramarital affairs as well as the conflicts we mentioned in the previous games.

The resolution of this game comes about through the communication of your anger or hurt at the specific incident that caused it. The sooner this hurt and anger is expressed, the sooner understanding and forgiving can be reached. Getting mad and getting over it is really much easier than getting even.

Guilt is the sense of dread or fear of consequences of a known wrongdoing. We have already explained that guilt is usually a very useful emotion in motivating healthy change. It may, however, become a part of a destructive game. In such cases, one partner may use the other's guilt as a weapon against him. In power struggles, for example, one partner may belittle the other by reminders of past misdemeanors.

The most positive emotion in life, of course, is love. Some emotions in marriage start out being loving but become confused by feelings of guilt or inadequacy and may result in the destruction of healthy sexual adjustment.

More than twenty years ago, I read a book by C. S. Lewis entitled *Four Loves.* In it, he defines the *agape* love of God or a parent for a child, the *phileo* love between brothers and sisters, the erotic love between husbands and wives, and the "Oh, you, too?" love in the sharing of exciting discoveries with a friend.

Perhaps in every close relationship there is something of all of these loves. When they get out of balance, however, there is likely to be trouble. In one marriage I know, the husband frequently acts like a child with his wife—not a playful child, in which she might join him, but a needy child, setting her up to play mother to him. He has done this intensively for a long time. Significantly, as this behavior has increased, their sex life has dwindled to nothing, largely because the mother-child love between them has unconsciously replaced their sexual love. Usually some guilt feelings are aroused by such a situation.

The same problem can arise when a husband and wife enter into the kind of competitive relationship (be it ever so loving and even useful in motivating them) they had with their brothers and sisters while growing up. Sooner or later, they may unwittingly feel like brother and sister. When this happens, as when one spouse feels parental, the brother-sister relationship may subtly erode the erotic feelings of an otherwise good marriage. It's wonderful to be friends, competitors, and certainly it's necessary to respond to one another's needs as parents, but do so carefully, limitedly, and always return to being primarily lovers.

Using Your Intellect

We have an understanding of physical facts and some emotional pitfalls and how to avoid them. Let's examine for a moment how to use your intellectual resources in enriching your sex life.

In chapter one, we discussed the fact that each person has only a limited amount of energy. This will vary with age, general health, emotional well-being, and other factors. But there is always a measurable limit. When a husband or wife expends too much of this life energy on the job, housekeeping, children, or personal activities, there simply may not be enough left for each other. There will, of course, be times of stress when ideal energy allotments cannot be achieved. Illness, financial burdens, and personal problems do come along to drain you and rob your energy for loving. When this happens to you, you need to do three things: 1. Recognize and admit to yourself that you are exhausted and form a plan to restore your energy. 2. Explain the situation to your spouse so he can avoid feeling neglected and sorry for himself. 3. Discipline yourself to plan and keep your values in their proper order of priority. An example of energy allocation and the importance of establishing priorities is exemplified in the following story.

Ken and Vickie had been married for ten years. They had three children. The oldest, a boy, was eight and becoming involved in various activities. Though Vickie did not have another career, she was fully occupied with taxiing David, playing with and reading to Donna, who was five, and could have been totally consumed by baby Jerrie, who was in the middle of those "terrible twos." She had no time to herself until the last child was in bed at nine o'clock.

Ken worked very hard, too, providing for the needs of his growing family and working for their future. But when he arrived home, he could relax in his easy chair, read the paper, and at best would grunt a response to the children's pestering. Usually he took a nap while they were being herded through their baths and to bed.

By then, Vickie could only collapse in a heap, but Ken was ready to talk or make love. He felt she should be more responsive since she was "at home all day." Vickie, an overly conscientious woman, felt she should be a "better wife" and took for granted that Ken knew how hard she worked and how tired she was. Fortunately, they began to communicate. When Ken got the information about her daily schedule, he understood her fatigue. And when Vickie knew it was all right to be human and ask for some help, gradually their family life improved. Ken rested while she fixed dinner and Vickie rested while he put the children to bed. They both had some time and energy for each other and the children began to get acquainted with their father. As an added benefit, Ken became a better role model for the children.

Love is a choice and a discipline. It demands that you climb out of the rut of old habits and their automatic expectations. To love is to explore what's right and good and cultivate it to be even better. To love is to be sensitive to what's wrong and painful and take the trouble and risk the honesty to figure out what to do about it—and together, work as long and hard as you need to make it right, good, and better!

Social Relationships

Before we conclude this chapter, we need to examine some facts about the sexual aspects of social situations. We have already seen that sexual desires may be aroused through social situations without ever exchanging a bit of love, or losing love for one's spouse.

Socially, outside the family, we in the Western world live with the belief that women and men (especially men!) are not supposed to show affection for a person of the same sex even as friends, because it may look as though they are homosexuals. It is socially acceptable, on the other hand, to be quite physically demonstrative to someone of the opposite sex, even if it causes hurt or jealousy to another person. Much social interaction involves subtle body language and innuendos that leave confusion at best, pain at worst, in people's minds and hearts.

Social relationships are for fun and friendship. It can be refreshing to be able to enter into a group as a straightforward, honest, caring person. There is a warm feeling in being able to hug friends —women or men—with a friendly "Hello" or a tender "Good-bye, take care!" without sexual implications. How comfortable to be free of the least twinge of guilt at some secret insinuation that would exclude my own spouse or someone else's!

Within the family, there are certain social customs that need your understanding. Your children need to see and feel the warmth and affection you have for one another as their parents. But they do not need to see or know about your sex life. Touching one another's erogenous zones or acting in an explicitly sexual manner in front of the kids is out of order.

Young children and adolescents have neither the experience nor the desire to deal with sexual matters. Their curiosity is easily aroused and they may become sexually stimulated, but they just don't know what to do about it. And they shouldn't have to do anything, because their energy needs to go into growing, playing, and learning. Later on, they may ask about your personal sex life, and it's appropriate to tell them if you are comfortable doing so.

In this same vein, children are uneasy when they see their parents nude. Little boys are vaguely attracted to their mothers and most little girls plan to grow up and marry their daddies. But they don't and shouldn't think of this in sexual terms. There's lots of time for that later when Mom is replaced by the girl down the street and Dad by the football star. Seeing parents nude often leaves children feeling inadequate, excited, and shy. So avoid it and teach the children to knock before entering the bathroom or your bedroom. Be sure to return the favor at their doors!

Be watchful of your children's relationships with each other. In chapter six, we will discuss this in more detail. But do understand that little children can very comfortably share a bathtub. It can, in fact, enable you to begin to explain sexual differences. But they will let you know when they want that stopped, and you need to listen and respond to that signal. Children will develop their own personalized balance in privacy and togetherness if they are allowed to do so.

The problem of sexual play or even exploration between brothers and sisters happens primarily: 1. when children see too much sexually stimulating behavior too soon and 2. when children are left too much to their own devices. Parents need not be snoopy, just around. When social life at home is happy, children will prefer to play around their parents. A healthy social life does begin at home—and usually ends up there, too!

Information From the Bible

Spiritually, information about sex and sexuality is very clear. Read again the beautiful story of the creation of Adam and Eve. Created for companionship, "They were both naked, the man and his wife, and were not ashamed" (Genesis 2:25).

Only when they had both disobeyed God and listened to the

voice of the serpent, who was more subtle than any other beast (Genesis 3:1), did Adam and Eve experience shame. They hid from God and sewed garments out of leaves.

Many people today blame God for inhibiting them and restricting their lives. This ancient story reveals that as false. It was not God but the voice of His enemy that misled Adam and Eve. In the restored state of redemption, married couples may be sexually free with one another, as were Adam and Eve.

God's commandments, "Thou shalt not commit adultery" and ". . . thou shalt not covet thy neighbour's wife . . ." (Exodus 20:14, 17) and several New Testament rules have a very important facet that many people do not think about. As I have come to understand God, He is a loving, protecting Creator. Jesus said, "Whom the Son sets free, shall be free indeed" (*see* John 8:36). I am convinced that these commands are for the good of people and not for their restriction. Being free, positively and constructively, means free to commit, grow, find peace and security—not free to search endlessly and neurotically for answers that are false and will never satisfy.

5

Sexual Responsibility

We have discussed sexual attitudes and how they affect our personal lives as well as their significant influence on teaching our children about sex. We have defined and clarified a great many facts about sex so that you will have a fund of information on which to draw as you teach. But it is also very important that you have a basic sense of responsibility about incorporating all this and actually getting down to the business of teaching your child.

A large part of responsibility involves living out of a series of choices and taking the consequences of those choices. A mature person must consider not only his own wishes or needs but must also be concerned with the needs of everyone involved in a particular situation.

Physically, we are responsible first of all to ourselves. Being honest and forthright about our sexuality and its expression is basic. Taking care of our own bodies and maintaining good health is vital.

Being aware of our emotions and how they influence our lives sexually is the second area of responsibility we will consider. Learning to control our emotions instead of letting them control us is part of growing up.

The third section of this chapter is about intellectual responsibility. Knowing those sometimes dry facts is essential to communicating meaningfully with our children. Being intellectually honest is important. It is easy to rationalize or kid ourselves into believing something is true when we know it isn't.

Responsibility to others in our interpersonal relationships is the fourth area of concern in this chapter. While we are not responsible for the actions of other adults, we are responsible for our behaviors and responses to them. And we certainly are responsible for teaching and training our children about sexuality.

Remembering that being whole people includes spiritual aspects of responsibility will be the last section. Seeing how the image of God, in which He created us, is portrayed in our lives is a powerful teaching tool for our children.

Physical Sexual Responsibility

Know Your Body

You are responsible for learning about your own body—both its anatomy and something of the way in which it functions. You also need to know the physical and functional differences between the male and female.

It is common for women in the week prior to a menstrual period to experience several pounds of weight gain, to feel tired, and to become irritable and gloomy. While she experienced this every month for many years, a friend of mine had never understood that this is a physiological process. Due to the level of certain hormones in the body that are a part of the menstrual cycle, the bodies of many women retain water. This fluid, collecting so quickly, causes most of the irritability through complex physical processes.

By understanding something of the entire mechanism of her body, my friend found out how to overcome most of her difficulty. She took extra rest time, cut down on her salt intake (since salt also tends to make our bodies store fluid) and consulted her doctor. He recommended some very safe medication and told her to limit her fluid intake. Not only was my friend a happier, more comfortable person but so were her husband and family. As her husband understood her physical problems, he became supportive rather than returning anger for her irritation.

Children, as they approach puberty, also go through dramatic physical changes. When they understand these, and especially when they know their parents understand, they can get through this difficult period with much more tranquility.

The Reverend Truman Dollar, with whom I coauthored *Teenage Rebellion,* told the poignant story of his own early-adolescent daughter. She was touchy and showed signs of slight estrangement or withdrawal from her family. Being people who greatly value family closeness, this was of some concern to her parents. As they talked together, it became clear to them that this girl was experiencing rapid physical and emotional changes. Ironically, though pubertal changes are relatively rapid, they do take place gradually enough that parents often do not focus really clearly on them. And rarely do they take time to do what these parents did. Pastor Dollar was the one who sat quietly with his daughter and described to her, simply, what was going on in her body. He told her that most young people during these months often feel emotions that are new and sometimes frightening. He reassured her that the tense times would pass, and she would again be comfortable with herself. Until then, both he and her mother would be available, understanding, and helpful in any way they could. The lovely young girl wept in her daddy's arms, tears of gratitude for the understanding she had craved. As you could imagine, both she and they weathered those stormy adolescent seas in good condition.

Take Care of Yourself

You are responsible for taking care of your body. We have learned that each of us has a limited amount of physical energy. Apportion your time to allow for enough sleep at night and occasional periods of rest during the day. Businesses and factories have discovered that work output and efficiency are increased by a short break in the middle of the morning and afternoon as well as a lunch period. This is true for the domestic engineers, otherwise known as "mothers," as well as people in jobs outside the home.

Taking breaks is not to be an excuse for laziness, however, because your body also needs exercise. Your job may provide adequate physical activity, but even the most active of jobs may limit you to one or a few sets of muscles. So running (walking, if you are like me!) and doing general body exercises will keep you in better condition. Be sure to do only the exercises your own body can tolerate and keep this part of yourself in balance with the rest of you.

Eating properly is a vital part of good health and energy. A dietician recently told me that she is concerned over the current "food fad" trend. Those who would eliminate meats, or carbohydrates, or any single nutritional element, may put their bodies in danger of malnutrition. The convenience of fast-food restaurants is very tempting in today's busy life. Be careful that you learn and practice a well-balanced diet. Eating together as a family offers a time to teach good dietary habits to children as well as providing a chance for regular communication.

Keep in Shape

You are responsible for keeping yourself physically attractive, clean, and well-groomed. Since home is a haven, it is a place to be comfortable. And to some people, being comfortable is being sloppy! A husband whose overweight stomach protrudes through an unbuttoned shirt and whose unshaven face feels like a brush, can hardly create romantic feelings in a trim wife who values neatness! Likewise, a wife who roams the house barefoot, braless, splitting the seams of last year's jeans, and with curlers in her hair, will almost certainly send her husband's gaze out the window, or worse!

A vicious cycle may be set in motion by failure to understand the importance of staying physically attractive. Denise finally consulted her family physician for help with her weight problem. After checking out all the possibilities, he found that she was a compulsive eater. Furthermore, Denise revealed that she recognized her tendency was to eat when her husband refused to participate in sexual relations with her. Unfortunately, his sexual interest and energy were much less than hers. Since she could not enjoy sex, eating, at least, gave Denise some sensual pleasure.

Don, her husband, was intolerant of Denise's eating habits and found her obesity repulsive. His sexual interest continued to decline while her eating habits became even worse. The vicious cycle was complete and tragically, this marriage ended in divorce. That divorce, as is true of most, would not have happened, had each of them, with help, been responsible enough to reach out to the other's needs and problems, rather than withdrawing and compensating.

Respond to Your Spouse's Needs

The story of Don and Denise also illustrates the need to sense and respond to each other's sexual needs. Had Don saved some energy, disciplined himself, and been less selfish, he could, to some degree at least, have increased his sexual functioning. His failure to even try to be more sexually responsive seems hostile as well as selfish and irresponsible. He may have needed counseling or medical attention. Recalling memories of their honeymoon, and other aids, could have helped to raise Don's sexual desire. But he refused. And Denise, helpless to get him to consider her sexual needs, could have sought counsel rather than drown her sadness and frustration in food. Failure to care about your spouse's sexual needs and ignoring them is sexually irresponsible. Doing nothing to change, for this couple, did everything to destroy a marriage.

Teach Your Child

As parents, we are responsible for our children's sex education and for teaching them, in turn, to be sexually responsible. Steven, our godson, used to come by our home frequently just to chat. As he became involved in dating, I asked him how he handled the loose morality of a large university campus. Steve's reply was classic—one of the most responsible attitudes I've ever heard. Before each date, he would look at himself in his mirror and say, "Steve, you take Terri's father's place with her this evening. Take care of her as he would and do nothing that would hurt either her or him." That self-lecture held Steve steady through many a tempting occasion.

Understanding VD

You are responsible for prevention and understanding of venereal diseases. Some years ago a friend was infected twice with gonorrhea by her own husband. He was one of those weak, undisciplined people who easily fell prey to his sexual impulses. For my friend, this was a humiliating experience, and certainly it was a cruel and selfish man who could carelessly put her through such difficulty.

You as parents need to know about venereal diseases for your own sake. But even more, you need to teach your adolescents about these diseases. They do not need to know in order to be frightened into sexual abstinence. Fear is not enough. They need to understand in order to be responsible. You may teach, discipline, and be ever so good an example, but some young people are just curious or rebellious enough that they are going to experiment sexually. I wish it were not true, but I know it is. And you need to know it, too! You need to know the signs of VD in order to protect your children. For a detailed explanation of VD *see* chapter ten.

Teenage Pregnancy and Birth Control

You are responsible for teaching your teenagers how to avoid unplanned pregnancy. Knowing that your teenage son or daughter may be sexually involved opens up a big area of responsibility for you parents as well as for the teenagers themselves. Many teens believe they will not be involved in a pregnancy, even though they are sexually active without using birth-control measures. One high-school girl told me she felt many of her friends believe that nothing serious or painful could ever happen to them because they have lived such sheltered lives. Her own parents had always taken care of and protected her. If she had problems, they solved them. When she was about to face unpleasant consequences for her irresponsibility, they usually rescued her. She felt that she lived a charmed life and believed that any major problem such as an unplanned pregnancy could never happen to her, no matter what she did.

One out of four births in a large midwestern city is to a teenage mother. Most of these are unmarried and totally dependent young women. A major factor in the teenage sexual revolution lies in the unwillingness of these young people to be responsible. In order to maintain some belief in their moral values, they avoid using contraceptives. In their minds, to use birth-control measures would be evidence that they planned to practice immorality.

The predicament in which this knowledge places you as parents is difficult. Should you give your daughter birth-control pills and teach your son about condoms? (You will find a discussion of birth-control measures in chapter eleven.) This is a weighty matter with grave implications. You need to responsibly consider all angles.

Most parents believe that to give a young person a contraceptive is like opening a door and inviting him or her to enter a sophisticated and exciting world of sexual activity. Few if any teenagers are ready for that world. Physical maturity is not complete until the age of nineteen or twenty and emotional and social maturity may require even more time. On the other hand, sexual promiscuity is everywhere. Avoiding discussions of such an issue may be the easy way out, but will not be beneficial to the children.

To further complicate this issue, medical personnel are legally allowed to provide birth-control measures to young people without their parents' knowledge. Perhaps it is better for you to know as much as possible about your child's sexual attitudes and any possible involvements, so you can guide him through all the complexities of his adolescence in a permissive and dangerous world.

Let me warn you that among the hundreds of teens with whom I have worked, lectures and demands have been fruitless. In fact, they often push the youngster directly into more rebellious behavior. What will work is to love and accept him while you are trying to understand and guide him. In chapter nine we will discuss in detail why young people become sexually active so prematurely.

It is true, with few exceptions, that such sexual activity in adolescents is based on real personal needs. As you reach out to these needs, you can help your special teen to grow in his self-awareness and sense of responsibility. With this sort of guidance, he will decide to wait for sex until he is ready for the commitment of marriage.

While it is true that most parental efforts to control teenagers' sexual activity fail to some extent, once in a while they are effective. A friend of mine was extremely troubled at the discovery of her sixteen-year-old daughter's sexual relationship with her boyfriend. At first all her commands and pleading failed to change the girl's decision to stay involved. At the mother's insistence, they both consulted a counselor. The girl discovered that much of her determination was really based on the fear of losing her boyfriend, rather than on love, as she had thought. She decided to stop the sex and develop other areas of their relationship. She realized that she and her boyfriend had missed many vital areas in getting to know each other as whole people because they had focused so exclusively on the physical aspects. In this case, had the mother not persisted, this girl would certainly have limited her relationship to mainly a sexual one.

A recent article quotes the alarming fact that roughly 50 percent of high-school girls have been sexually involved prior to graduation. The decision to advise your children about birth control is yours. You need to know, however, the degree of your child's sexual involvement and act accordingly.

Emotional Sexual Responsibility

Being emotionally responsible means 1. Making the choice about my own feelings. 2. Thinking clearly, discussing differences honestly, and getting through misunderstandings, hurts, or anger with others, directly and as soon as possible. 3. Being sensitive to my spouse, child, or friend, so I can respond to his needs and feelings with support. 4. Avoiding any words or actions that I believe may hurt another person. 5. Remembering to ask another what he needs, if anything, emotionally. 6. Clarifying communications, verbal or nonverbal, to avoid misunderstandings.

All of these rules for emotional responsibility converge on your sex life because they keep you emotionally close to one another. There is nothing like a stack-up of resentments, or a habit of game playing with all those bad feelings, to put a barrier between you in bed. Choosing to avoid negative feelings, you can build good, loving, trusting feelings into as close a relationship as you want.

With your children, too, you need to keep warm and positive feelings. If you worry over them too much, they will become convinced that something is wrong with them. If you are critical and angry too much, they will give up and quit trying. They will retaliate in anger and rebellion. If you nag at them, they will resist you, quietly but surely. If you lecture too much, they will develop calloused eardrums and tune you out.

But I can assure you that if you love them absolutely and show and tell them that you do, they will love you back. Have you ever tried to stay angry at someone who persists in loving you? I'll bet you can't do it for long. If you brag about your child, honestly and simply, he will learn to know he is a worthwhile person, and he will be motivated to do even better. If you train and discipline him when he is small, he will become someone of whom to be truly proud. If you are as consistent as possible, your child will come to know what to expect and that will give him security.

Intellectual Sexual Responsibility

There are many times when I simply don't like to face the facts. I know how I want something to be, but I cannot always make it that way. And therein lies the issue of intellectual responsibility. Some months ago, I had an absolutely terrible day at work—the worst I'd endured for quite a while. But I had to cope in order to help others cope, and to help the institution, where I carry a great deal of responsibility, to function smoothly. On that particular day, I managed to make it by picturing the end of the day. I would go home, ask my husband to put his arms around me, and perhaps I would even cry on his shoulder.

At the end of that day, I walked into my home just ready to

collapse in the proverbial heap. Fortunately, just short of falling, I took a look at my husband. The entire dining-room table was covered with the papers that are necessary to prepare an income-tax return. It was due in a few days, and I knew immediately that he needed my shoulder (if he were to admit it) more than I needed his that evening. My mind slipped into gear and figured a way we could both work out our needs.

This was an emotional versus an intellectual need, but the principle applies sexually, too. When one's sexual feelings and needs conflict with the other's, someone has to yield. Keeping such an issue on an intellectual plane and resolving it with logic will keep you sexually close.

If one or the other spouse makes a habit over a period of time of avoiding sexual relations, you need to deal with it. Find out together why one is losing interest in sex. It is difficult to explore such a sensitive area without blaming or defending. Being responsible, however, means that you can choose to discuss the issue calmly and with empathy for each other.

I can hear some of you saying, "What's all this emphasis on sex about, anyway? Is it really so important?" If both husband and wife believe it's not so important, if they are close to each other and not feeling sexually neglected or frustrated, then it's not an issue. But when one's needs are ignored or unknown to the other, sexually or in any other way, there's something wrong with that relationship that needs correcting. Even if it means swallowing a bit of pride and admitting that you need help to enable you to renew your sexual relations, it will bring such rewards that you will agree it was well worth it.

Your intellect enables you to control your emotions. The stories of *Camelot* and *Doctor Zhivago* are examples of a highly romantic concept. This concept says that in spite of love and the vows of marriage, when someone new (or an old love) comes along, people may fall madly, passionately in love and cannot help themselves. They say, "This thing is bigger than both of us." And that, I believe, is a selfish excuse for intellectually refusing to control one's emotions. You can choose to control your emotions, and it is your responsibility to do so.

You are also responsible to control the intensity with which you express your feelings. While it is of the utmost importance not to deny or hide your emotions, it is equally important that you do not allow feelings to erupt with volcanic devastation. I understand that you may simply be an explosive person and you may feel that people should learn to accept you just as you are. But explosive people can learn to know when pressures are building up and they can prevent explosions by expressing themselves early before things get out of control. Certainly emotions are powerful, and they keep life interesting, but you can and must be even stronger than they are. My three-part plan for dealing with feelings may bear repeating: 1. Express precisely how you feel. 2. Determine why you feel it. 3. Decide what you can and will do about it.

The reason for using your intellect and will to control your emotions is, obviously, the prevention of hurt feelings. Many people wrongly believe that what is said in anger is what people really mean—not the things they say when they are calm. I want you to know that this is certainly not true! When people become strongly emotional, they revert to childish patterns of expressing themselves. Children who are hurt or angry usually instinctively hurt back, and they have an uncanny ability to know what will hurt the other person. What they say in anger, therefore, is said for its effect in getting even, and may have no resemblance to their honest, rational thinking. Adults do not lose that ability or the habit of getting even unless they discipline themselves and work hard to change it.

So if you are an exploder, you need to do two things. First, learn to control yourself, and second, while you are in the process of forming the new habit, be sure to explain afterward what you really did and did not mean to say. Be sure you know the difference between "control" and "denial." The latter is dishonest and pretends that you do not feel what, in fact, you do feel. Control is expressing feelings in a thoughtful and constructive way.

Many people confuse feelings and ideas, but it is important to separate the two. When someone says, "I feel like ———," or "I feel that ———," be quite sure that what's coming next is not a feeling but an idea. But if the comment is, "I feel sad," or "I feel angry when————," then, clearly, you are hearing a feeling. The reason you need to know the difference is so that you can respond accurately. Opinions or ideas usually need discussion and may require some decision. Feelings, on the other hand, need caring, or defusing, or some emotional response. When these are kept clear, you will find it easier to stay loving and positive with one another.

Social Sexual Responsibility

Being sexually responsible socially certainly is a difficult assignment in today's Western world. From bumper stickers to major books, the philosophy is taught that sexual freedom and pleasure are goals to pursue. One bumper sticker I see regularly says, IF IT FEELS GOOD, DO IT! Complete self-indulgence is a way of life that many people pursue.

Guidelines for Social Situations

In your social interactions outside the home, you may well think of these guidelines:

Act with other people in social or business situations as you would act if your spouse or even your children were present.

A friend of mine is a woman in a highly competitive business dominated by men. She is friendly and at times seems slightly flirtatious in her manner. She told me that some men take advantage of this friendliness and make it subtly clear to her that they will give her their company's business if she will give them sexual favors. She has been able to avoid capitulating to their pressures because it is easier for her to resist than to endanger her children's respect for her.

Protect your self-respect and that of your family, and be responsible enough to help protect others from their own sexual impulses. That involves being conscious of any sexual inferences being exchanged. It may mean refusing to laugh at dirty jokes, and with some people, it may mean shaking hands instead of giving a friendly hug. It takes great sensitivity to one's own feelings as well as others' to know where to set limits—and self-control to stick with these limits.

When I was in high school, I was able to get a coveted job as cashier in a restaurant in our small town. It was during World War II, and there were many servicemen who came through our town. The owner of this lovely restaurant complimented me highly when he said he valued my ability to be friendly with these men without being "cheap." Now, more than then, I understand what a problem it is to find and keep that fine balance.

Avoid categorizing people sexually or in any other way. Whether male or female, respect them and accept them as individuals.

Stereotypes such as "male chauvinist" or "women's libber" may become ammunition in the warfare between the sexes in our Western society. Patricia had been severely emotionally hurt by her father and had married a man who compounded that hurt. She had unconsciously categorized all males as threatening and included her son in that group. He was beginning to develop emotional problems when she realized what she was doing. Fortunately, she began to accept her son as an individual and loved him back to health.

Guidelines for Family Interaction

Within the family, there are also some useful and important social guides.

Treat your spouse with respect and kindness, not only for his sake but also as an example for your children.

There is an interesting phenomenon that I have observed repeatedly. When one parent treats the other with disrespect, the children may imitate that attitude. But they usually lose respect for the discourteous parent as well.

Respect yourself and expect your family to respect you, too. I have seen patient, kind parents who allowed their children to insult and disobey them regularly. Though spirited children will test the limits parents set as far as they can, they want parents to hold firm at some point. Children often feel guilty when they are allowed to get by with disrespectful treatment of their parents, so you need to demand respect.

Janet is an example of such a situation. From infancy, she had found ways to get the better of her mother. When she was told not to eat candy before dinner, she waited until her mother left the room and ate it anyway. On the rare occasions when her mother restricted her to her room for hurting a playmate, she would cry and act sorry enough to be allowed outside, where she continued abusing her friends. When she became older, she learned to threaten her mother with, "If you don't let me spend the night with Susie, I'll run away!" To avoid Janet's anger and manipulation, her mother gave in to her demands so often that their positions were completely reversed. Eventually, Janet required intensive psychiatric care because she could not handle the responsibility of the power her mother gave her.

Respect your children as human beings, and show this by listening to their ideas, responding to their feelings, and praising their achievements. Showing respect for children (or any other person) means that a parent must know what that particular child's best behavior or performance may be and then require that that best be done. Sexual respect for children means that parents should respect their child's privacy as well as their own. They should not tease young children about "boyfriends" or "girl friends." It is tempting for little children to want to grow up too soon. Especially in their mode of dress, girls may push this earlier and more forcefully than boys. Seeing prepubertal girls in bras and high heels (apart from playing dress-up at home) is a sad sight because it symbolizes a premature loss of childhood. Yet many parents allow this or even promote it. There is such a long time to be adult and the responsibilities of adulthood are heavy. I believe children should stay free as long as is reasonably possible and gradually accept responsibilities proportionate to their ages.

Teaching responsibility to your children and educating them sexually is primarily your job as a parent. There is much arguing and fighting about sex education in the schools. Many sincere Christians fear schools will mislead their children in sexual values, yet they fail to teach them at home. I feel grateful for every school administrator and teacher who is willing to try to assume such a heavy responsibility in the place of parents. They need your help and support. Nevertheless, this is our responsibility as parents. We are the only ones who can teach our values to our children in the way and at the time we want it to be done. Children are going to learn about sex. If we as parents do not teach them, they may learn from each other or from "street talk." If we do not shoulder our responsibility, it's not fair to be upset with teachers who are doing the best they can.

Spiritual Sexual Responsibility

One of the problems with today's humanistic philosophy is the elimination of spiritual considerations. When people live for the satisfaction of sensual or physical cravings only, they lose the spiritual component that completes their true humanness. God created man in His image, and we are specifically told that God is a spirit. So it is ultimately in our spiritual nature that we are like God. It seems that the cultivation of that component of our being, then, should be of the utmost importance.

Throughout history and in many different cultures and religions, the growth of spiritual values has prompted "ascetic" living, or the withdrawing from social and sexual relationships into an isolated life. This seems to be the opposite swing of the pendulum from the hedonistic or sensual life-style of permissiveness.

Seeing sexual relationships in their right perspective, then, involves the avoidance of either hedonism or asceticism. Maintaining a clear understanding of the true meaning of sex is essential. It is an expression of intimacy and love, or a means of conceiving a child to enrich the love of wife and husband. It is, as the Bible says beautifully, a symbol of the closeness we enjoy with Jesus Christ. It is only when this perspective is lost that sex becomes distorted.

As parents, you need to understand these facts for your own fulfillment, and you need to teach them to your children. They need to know that God asks nothing of His children except that which is for their very highest good. When God commanded,

"Thou shalt not commit adultery" (Exodus 20:14) and "Flee fornication . . ." (1 Corinthians 6:18), He did that for our ultimate good
and not to restrict our pleasure. I believe He knew how unbalanced
people might become when such sexual pursuits were unre-
strained. The case for sexual responsibility and obedience to God's
laws concerning sexual relationships is no exception to this principle of our good being His greatest concern.

When I was a student, a literature professor taught me a basic
concept of what must be present to create a masterpiece. Whether
that work is music, art, drama, or literature, one of the essentials
of greatness is the use of a repetitive theme or pattern. That theme,
varying and recurring throughout the work, gives the receiver a
sense of familiarity. The work can be remembered and understood.

God's creation, and His plan for the life and interaction of the
entire system of creation, is such an amazing masterpiece. But the
pattern of closeness between parents, shared by parents and child,
among brothers and sisters, among friends, and finally, spiritually
between a person and Himself, certainly portrays one part of
God's masterpiece!

As each one of us gets to know and accept ourselves, our
strengths, and inevitable weaknesses, we have the cornerstone of
healthy sexual responsibility. As we add the acceptance and understanding of a spouse, there is another part of the foundation for
living. Responsibly conceiving and raising children adds a third
component. The four corners of a great foundation are completed
as we learn to live responsibly with others. The strength throughout the building of our lives is the power and presence of God in
all of our being.

Part Two

Parental Training

6

How to Teach Your Baby About Sex

Please go no further in this book if you have not understood and found some agreement with the first chapters. If you do not know that good sex education begins with your attitudes, depends on the accuracy of your information, and is only learned in an atmosphere of responsibility, you will be more than likely to endanger the success of the actual teaching process!

Your parents may have failed miserably in teaching you about sex, but you can do better. Even if you feel you have already failed, you can correct your mistakes. The secret to good education is to encourage curiosity and to respond to and satisfy that curiosity in increments. A child's questions need to be answered simply and specifically. The following story illustrates this point.

Jimmy came home from kindergarten and startled his mother with the question "Where did I come from?" His mother had been expecting just such a question, and she explained the facts of life to Jimmy in detail. He listened patiently until she finished, but still looked puzzled. "But Mommy," he asked, "where did I come from? Nancy came from New York and Johnny came from Iowa. Where did I come from?"

You can see how essential it is to determine what your child really wants to know and respond to that.

Effective Teaching Methods

Besides verbal teaching and responses, there are other effective ways to teach your child about sex.

The way you most meaningfully communicate is by your own attitudes and beliefs. The "how" of sex education becomes an automatic transmission from you to your children. There are other ideas, however, that may help you.

Become, if you aren't, a lover of nature. Take your children for hikes in a park or out in a natural area such as woods or a pasture. Show them insect eggs, caterpillars, cocoons, and butterflies. They will love the incomparable blue of a robin's eggshell. Baby animals, tadpoles, and fish are all exquisite pieces of the puzzle that depicts life and how it begins. And that is part of sexuality.

Many people dislike reading, but to really teach your children, you need to read. Gaining your own information can hardly be adequate without reading, and sharing books and pictures with your children will give them significant advantages. First, they will gain information; second, sharing it with you will develop a happy intimacy that is a child's real security; third, they will early develop a habit of curiosity, learning, and mental growth that will extend through their entire lives.

Use television to teach your children about sex. Many thoughtful people despair about TV and its explicit portrayal of violence and sex. But it is there and your children will be exposed to it in one way or another. Watching television with your children will provide the opportunity to distinguish positive from negative values in many areas of life.

Verbally share your ideas and observations with your children. Though my parents did not have an opportunity for much formal schooling, they discussed values and ideas around the dinner table regularly. Many of my own values have been sifted out of those conversations, which I vividly recall, even now.

The Right Time

When to tell your child about sex is also a sensitive issue. In today's world, children at an unusually tender age are aware of highly sophisticated sexual facts. Your children in kindergarten may hear comments that bear explaining. Each child is very different in his sexual interest, awareness, and comprehension. Perhaps these suggestions will help:

Think of starting at the birth of your child and make sex education an ongoing process. That takes away the pressure of staging a time, getting as much said as you can, and getting through with it. That is definitely the wrong philosophy!

I will never forget the red-faced, squirming discomfort I felt when my mother told me the "facts of life and masturbation." At least she did tell me and I appreciate that, because many parents just never get around to that. I must say, however, that my best sexual attitudes came from seeing her with my father in those tender times. And seeing baby chicks hatch and newborn baby animals reflected in my father's twinkling brown eyes, made the creation of life a warm reality.

Be alert and listen to each child's interests. A question or even an inquiring glance may be your clue that it is time for another episode in telling your child about sex. Remember to give him only what he is ready to hear. Sometimes, out of our own nervousness, we talk too much. It's better to talk a little, as simply and directly as the child can comprehend, and invite further discussion later.

When you have a child who doesn't ask, you do have a problem. For some reason, there are such youngsters who focus their attention on other aspects of life or are unusually shy. It is with such a child that a nature hike can be useful, or a simple question such as, "Jim, I was thinking the other day, that you've never seemed to wonder about babies and sexual matters. Do you have any questions?" If not, simply invite him to ask you whenever such questions arise. Giving such a child any age-appropriate book that he may read in private may help, too.

When a sexual experience in life happens, that is a good time to discuss it and it can be very useful as a teaching tool. A new baby in the family, a litter of kittens on your block, or a television special may make a wonderfully natural occasion for teaching about sex. You may need to initiate the conversation with your child by asking him a question or explaining a situation.

My brother, a farmer, tried very hard to teach his children good sexual attitudes and information. He explained simply and kindly the answers to their childish questions. One winter evening he was in the barn helping a mother sheep deliver a little lamb. In his intentness he became vaguely aware of a shadow in the doorway. As he looked up, he saw his seven-year-old daughter gazing wide-eyed at the ever-miraculous process of birth. With evident pleasure and some relief, she said, "It's just exactly like you said it was, Daddy!" She had heard his teaching and now she knew it was so. Frankly, I feel sorry for city dwellers who have few opportunities to teach and learn from nature!

Whenever and however you teach your children the facts of life, there is one deadline you must beat! That deadline is the onset of puberty. By the time your son or daughter is capable of conception, they need to know how pregnancy occurs, when it can take place, and they need to have a deep sense of responsibility. Few experiences in my life have been as sad as witnessing the cutting short of carefree youth by an unwanted and premature pregnancy. There is no happy solution to this problem, once it is a reality, and the only answer is prevention.

You will make some mistakes in this whole teaching process. But the only unforgivable mistake is silence. To discuss, listen, guide, and teach your children is primarily your responsibility, as parents.

Now let's think about how you can (and do) teach even a tiny child about sex.

Physical Aspects

A child's first picture of himself is seen through his parents' eyes. Even physically, this is true. Babies see very poorly at birth; they are drawn at first to focus on bright, shiny things, such as parents' eyes. Look at the dark center of someone's eye (the pupil) closely, and you can see yourself reflected there. Probably a baby sees only the brightness that shines back from his parents' eyes, but certainly the way he sees himself as a person is just as the parent sees him.

Teaching Your Baby

There are special reflections of your opinion of your infant that he will come to see in your face and the way you handle him. One rather squeamish young mother actually gagged as she medicated her baby's umbilical cord and changed his dirty diaper. While I give her *A* for effort in keeping on with his care in spite of her distaste, I often wonder what message that spoke to him about his body. Most parents are not so squeamish as that, but a great many grimace or use some body language of disgust in the physical care of an infant.

Picture yourself, if you will, as a brand-new father or mother changing a baby boy's bowel-stained diaper. Before this unpleasant mess is cleaned up, and even while you are bent over his miniature body to do it, he has the nerve to spray you with urine, as well! It would take a saint or an angel to refrain from what many parents do: howl with rage at such an insult. Now imagine the innocent, helpless infant who can only be amazed and confused at this response to his perfectly natural body functions.

Since they are anatomically so close, the baby's excretory areas (the rectum and urethra) are, to him, a part of his sex organs. When parents react with displeasure or disgust, he learns early that this part of his body is distasteful and may even be shameful.

I would be foolish to tell you that you must learn to enjoy the odor of a baby's bowel movement or the feel of that unexpected urinary shower! But since these functions are evidence of a normal, healthy body, I can reassure you that you may balance that distaste with gratitude for the health of that child. With effort and time, you can even attend to the toilet care with as much grace and dignity as any other demands of your infant, such as feeding or rocking.

A young mother I know well was once complaining to her husband about her frustrations with dirty diapers, formulas, and laundry. His answer, as he gently hugged her, was, "If we didn't have to go through all this, maybe we wouldn't appreciate or enjoy them so much later." I might add that he was not saying that from his easy chair, but from the nursery, where he helped her in these duties!

Physically, parents also teach a baby to accept his body as they react to his self-discovery. From time immemorial, mothers have delightedly sung some version of these nursery rhymes to their babies, complete with appropriate motions:

> Head bumper
> Eye winker
> Tom tinker
> Nose smeller
> Mouth eater

or

> This little piggy went to market.
> This little piggy stayed at home.
> This little piggy had roast beef.
> This little piggy had none.
> This little piggy cried, "Wee, wee, wee!"
> All the way home.

A baby's crow of delight at this method of learning his little anatomy is worth a call to doting grandparents! But when the little angel discovers his or her genitals, quite another response is likely! I have seen parents slap the hands of a baby for such a normal motion as touching the penis or the vagina and then quickly encase the "embarrassing" genitals in a tight diaper. How can an infant understand such a reaction? And how can he grow to believe that a loving, wise God made all of him?

More thoughtful parents may just as hurriedly, but more gently, distract the child's attention with a toy. The message, though milder in its impact, is similar.

Let me suggest that you try instead to allow the infant to explore the genital areas, just as he does his nose and ears. Tell him or her the name of the penis or vagina with the same pleasure you show when he learns the other parts of his body. You will find that after only a short time, the baby's interest will focus elsewhere. He will not become preoccupied with his genitals any more than his hands or nose, unless you do. Your comfortable attitude toward the infant's genitals will convey to him a calm, happy acceptance of his whole body that will be a lasting benefit to him. As you learn this natural attitude toward your baby's body, you will be growing more relaxed and confident in your ability to verbally speak to your older child about sexual issues. Your comfort with this usually uneasy "chore" of sex education can grow to a point where it is remarkably easy and natural.

Now you have overcome your distaste and can take care of baby's toilet needs. You are no longer horrified or embarrassed when he or she touches the genital area. There is a third area of importance in a young child's physical sex education that relates to toilet training. Lest this sound alarmingly Freudian, let me assure you it is not. Remember that the child's genitals and the areas of excretion are so close that, to him or her, they are one and the same. When toilet training is started too soon, before a child is able to voluntarily control the muscles involved in these body functions, he simply cannot respond. Such control is rarely possible until two to three years of age. When parents do not understand these facts, they may believe a child is stubborn and needs punishing. There are always relatives or friends who had *their* babies trained by the time they were a year old! While this occasionally happens, it is probably the parent who is trained to catch the excretory habits of an unusually adaptable and regulated child rather than the child's being trained.

Harshness, threats, and punishment may eventually work in toilet training a child. But there is a price tag attached. It includes the development of certain emotional problems: fear, anxiety, and later on, anger. All too often, these are expressed unconsciously through sexual hang-ups. So don't be in a hurry to get your child out of diapers. I have never seen a healthy child wearing diapers to kindergarten, but I have seen children wetting and soiling their clothes in school because of fear and tension. Take your time in teaching. Explain and show the child how to use the toilet and be proud when he does!

The fourth aspect of physically teaching your baby about sex involves simply holding and cuddling your child. Most babies instinctively nestle into their parents' arms. They will usually show contentment, and when they have been fussy may grow quiet at being held. They relax to the rocking motion. I strongly believe that every child needs to be rocked by his parents. When such holding is both strong and relaxed, babies experience security and enjoyment of physical intimacy. As they grow, babies will love to feel tickling and blowing on their skin, and later they love tossing and rough play, as long as they experience this with strong adult handling.

Singing to babies is another soothing and enjoyable means of helping them to enjoy close physical contact. Making up tunes or modifying old nursery rhymes to include the baby's name helps him to feel important.

Whatever you may do that transmits to your baby a sense of the warmth of your unconditional love and his unique importance to you will be laying a foundation of self-confidence for his life.

There is another useful way to give little children a natural lesson in anatomical differences. That is to have a young son and daughter bathe together. While playing in the water, they will notice that he has a penis and she doesn't, in a casual, nonthreatening way. Be sure to spend some time near them so they may ask you about the differences. And again, if they don't ask, casually mention the fact that they are made differently and explain that that is how God created people to be. Tell them that someday boys may become daddies and girls may become mommies and that's why they need to be different. They will listen and then start splashing water on each other. But they will have the seeds of truth planted in their minds. As they reach the age of six or seven, by the way, children will inevitably ask, "Do I have to bathe with her [or him] anymore?" That is your signal that your growing child is ready for some privacy, and he needs to be granted that.

By the age of three, most children are talking quite fluently and understand a great deal more than most parents can believe. They are likely to start asking questions about many things. When they are about four years of age, most children drive their parents to distraction by constantly asking, "Why?" Be sure you take time to look at your child as you answer all of these questions the best way you can. Your availability and interest will keep the communication lines open for more questions later.

Explaining Pregnancy

Usually by the age of three or four, a new sibling is on the way, or the child will see a pregnant mother of a friend. If your child asks why your (or her) tummy is big, it is a wonderful chance to verbally teach him the elemental story of the creation of a new life. Tell him something such as this: "A tiny egg within the mother has been joined with a similar object, called a sperm, from the father. This special egg, so small that we can't even see it without a big magnifying glass, grows ever so slowly in a place in the mother's body that is called a 'womb.' The womb is like a tiny room where this growing egg is safe, fed by the mother's body until it is ready to be born. By only a few weeks of age, this amazing egg has begun to develop into a baby with tiny arms, legs, a body, and a head, just like yours. Before three months, the baby has fingers and toes and looks like a little you.

"Inside of this tiny baby there are all the things you have: a heart, lungs to breathe with, a stomach to hold food, and all the parts of the body that keep us alive and healthy. While these things are all there so early, the baby needs to grow lots more before it is ready to leave this safe little nest. It is amazing how God made our bodies, because as this baby starts out, the nest is about the size of your fist. But as the baby grows, the nest grows, too, until the baby is ready to be born and weighs about seven pounds or even more. Most babies are about twenty inches long. [You may show a curious child about how big that is.]

"We don't know exactly how the mother and baby both know it is time for it to be born, but it is about nine months after the tiny egg began to grow that birth happens. Maybe the baby feels too closed in. Maybe the mother's womb, or nest, feels too stretched. At any rate, the nest begins to squeeze itself a little— like you squeeze your fist. The mother can't make this happen. It just happens by itself, because that's the way God planned it for us long ago when He created our world and us.

"That squeezing makes a feeling that tells a mother her baby will soon be born, so she goes to the hospital. Babies could be born at home, but it is easier and safer to be where there are doctors and nurses who can help the mother and take care of the baby while she rests for a few days. As the nest continues to squeeze and rest, squeeze and rest, the baby is slowly pushed downward from the mother's tummy into the tube called a vagina that leads from the womb to the outside world through an opening between the mother's legs. There is an opening to the womb called the 'cervix,' and it slowly opens to let the baby into the vagina and at last through to the wide world where we live.

"All of this beautiful process takes several hours, maybe half a day or more. And it makes the mother quite tired because sometimes with all that squeezing and stretching, she gets pretty uncomfortable. That is why she needs to go to the hospital —not because she is seriously ill. If the mother is too uncomfortable, the doctor will give her some medication to help her feel better."

As you tell this story to your child, you will want to be aware of several things. First, be sure that your telling this conveys your sense of joy and wonder at the amazing process it is. Be careful to avoid any undue emphasis on the pain or risks involved. That's why I suggest the terms *uncomfortable* and *squeezing* rather than *painful* or *labor.*

Next, be watchful of your child's response to this narrative. He may be ready for only a part of this story at a time, or he may listen in rapt attention. Give him only what he can handle at the time. When he starts to look around, tell him this is a continued story and when he wants to hear the next part, he may ask for it. This avoids boredom and best of all, it sets the pattern for recurrent teaching and sharing about sex and all sorts of other important issues.

Notice your child's facial expression. If you see worry or pleasure, stop and ask him what he's thinking about. Give him a chance to ask questions as you talk. Children learn much more when they discuss topics with us rather than just listening to us lecture. Any questions your three- or four-year-old may ask, you can answer. Most answers can be short and simple. A preschooler is rarely interested in a detailed account of sexual intercourse! He may want to know, however, how it is that the father's sperm gets inside the mother's body. A simple statement that sperm is made inside the daddy's scrotum and goes through his penis into the mother's vagina will make that clear.

If you aren't certain about some answers, it is quite all right to say that you don't have that information but you will find out. While children at this age do believe parents know everything, they need to learn, and can accept, that you really don't. If you remember to find out and tell them, however, they will learn that you are reliable, that their concerns are important, and that you care. And that's even more important a lesson than sex education.

At times, a child may ask to see his mother's vagina or his father's scrotum. It is rarely wise to grant such a request because the normal anatomy is very different from that of a mother during the birth process which is being described and because most people prefer some privacy about their bodies. A verbal description will usually satisfy a child, or a simple diagram may be shown. You will find such a diagram in this book or in your own library or encyclopedia.

If you have missed the chance to relate these facts to your child while he is small and more curious, do not despair. Here is a suggestion for you. Look for a new opportunity. Looking means to observe your child in all situations, but for the purpose of teaching about sex, be especially aware of situations that may arouse some interest or questions in sexual matters. A new litter of kittens or puppies in the neighborhood, news of a new baby in your community, even a television show or carefully selected book, will serve this need. Now it is your turn to ask the child if he understands how babies come to be and how they are born. Invite him to let you tell him at a convenient time, or to read him a book. Prior to school age, most children love having parents read a book to them. You may choose to read these paragraphs or to select from your local library a book such as *The Wonderful Story of How You Were Born,* by Sidonie M. Gruenberg, with its child-oriented pictures.

Always be sure that you are comfortable before you approach the subject of sex. Children are highly sensitive to adult emotions, and your child will almost certainly shy away from this topic if you feel uneasy. Talk about the issues of the moment with your spouse or a friend, rehearse in front of a mirror, or do whatever you can to become as relaxed and natural as possible.

Emotional Aspects

A young child learns to feel ashamed, afraid, guilty, or angry when parents "miss the boat" by demonstrating these attitudes in their teaching about sex. But when parents remember to practice their wholesome attitudes and give information in a consistently responsible way, the strong foundation of self-esteem is formed and a loving, trusting bond between parent and child is secured.

As the young child grows, sexual emotions continue to unfold. By the age of two or three, many children begin to react in fear when they see a nude adult. An adult's stature alone may be awesome to a little child, but the sight of adult genitals or breasts may by their visibility increase that awe to fear. They can only wonder why they have no breasts and why daddy's penis is larger than theirs. At this age they have no vocabulary with which to ask. Quite early, children have some sense of their own and their parents' sexuality. They also have prime evidence of their power-lessness and usually feel insignificant, according to Leontine Young's perceptive book *Life Among the Giants.*

Because of this evidence, it seems advisable for families to avoid nudity during this time in their child's life and for some time afterward. You as a parent may simply prefer some privacy for yourself. This can be had by setting up a few rules. Young children can be taught to knock on a closed door and wait for the parent to get a robe before opening it. It's not a bad idea to teach young-sters to respect others' territory. Should a child enter the room without remembering to knock, please don't panic and yell. Sim-ply ask him to hand you a towel or a robe and remind him of the rule to knock. The child wants to be near you because he loves or needs you. If you respond to that as a compliment, the invasion of your privacy becomes unimportant.

When parents have mistakenly become angry and punished a child over innocent, childhood sexual discoveries or toilet training, certain emotional responses may be expected. These usually are anger and defiance, withdrawal and fear, or secretiveness and guilt.

When a child is punished for curiosity about his genitals, he may become preoccupied with them. He may learn to masturbate compulsively but secretly, fostering guilt and fear, or he may become so afraid of his genitals that adult sexual pleasure is impossible.

The problem in sex education of the young child is not his curiosity or exploring of his sex organs. The problem relates to what such actions symbolize to the parents. It is out of the loss of their created innocence that they misinterpret such actions and overreact to the child. This need not take place, parents, if you remember what you have read.

As an adult, Julie developed anxiety attacks; her heart would pound and she had to breathe heavily. She was subject to ulcers and often had nightmares or trouble getting to sleep. Sometimes she would cry or rage over minor happenings. During therapy, she recalled that as a very young child her father had repeatedly demanded to "check" her genitals during a bath or for no known reason. Being a shy child by nature, Julie was intensely ashamed and fearful of these inspections. She pleaded with her father to let her alone, but he insisted it must be done.

Julie's helplessness, added to her embarrassment, left indelible scars in her mind and her emotions. When adult situations occurred that revived these old memories, the rage and panic born of her sense of helplessness would return. The emotions overflowed into other areas of her life besides sexual ones. Early-childhood problems do leave deep scars. While they can be healed, they are much more easily prevented.

How can you make matters right if you have already mishandled your child's early sex education? First of all, feel comforted in the fact that you have lots of company. In a lecture to a large class of university students recently, I asked how many of them felt their parents had taught them adequately about sexual matters. Only one hand went up. Only a few believed their parents had actually taught them anything about sex. And this has been a relatively sexually "liberated" generation of parents.

You may be one of those parents, unable to lay even the foundation for healthy sex education because of your excessive inhibitions or lack of information. If you practice what you have been reading, with the proper attitudes and feelings, you can now discuss and think about sexual issues without either embarrassment or excitement. You can use appropriate rather than crude or vulgar terms in discussing sexual areas comfortably.

Have you read and talked about your body and your spouse's so that your information is adequate? Have you made this information so completely yours that you can translate it into terms even your young child can understand? Are you willing to share that information with your child when he asks? If he is past asking, will you find a time and place to tell him in appropriate ways what he needs to know? If so, your rating as a good sex educator goes up!

Being responsible about sexual issues may well mean that you need to apologize for past mistakes or omissions. As soon as children are old enough to understand, they love to hear stories about their earliest babyhood. You may use this interest to relate a story that includes an episode of unfair punishment or any mistake that troubles you. You needn't tell all the sorry details, but out of the story can come a healing of your own troubled heart as your child, so naturally forgiving, lets you know he loves you even with your faults. And when you tell stories that involve sexual matters, you may explain the way you wish you had handled the situation.

At any rate, start where you are now and do it right from here on. Use your wholesome attitudes, your good information, and your sense of responsibility to make your child's sex education great from now on. No one else can teach your child what you want him to know, so don't wait for school, Sunday school, or the neighborhood kids to do it for you!

Intellectual Aspects

Mentally, the young child will build a belief system remarkably like that of his parents. If they believe men are superior to women, so will the child. If they see women as domineering or controlling, the child will tend to agree. Beliefs grow out of attitudes and behaviors which may often be so habitual that we are actually not aware of them. As parents, therefore, stop and think about what you are teaching your child. Take inventory of your beliefs and see if your attitudes and ideas are consistent. Be sure your information is accurate.

By school age there are five attitudes your child needs to understand if he is to be a sexually healthy person: 1. He needs to know that he is a beautiful child and that his imperfections only add to his uniqueness as a masterpiece created by God and nurtured by you. 2. He needs to understand that every other person is also intended to be beautiful and unique and, therefore, to be respected as he respects himself. 3. He needs to know some of the physical differences between boys and girls and some facts about how babies are conceived and born. 4. He needs to have learned to respect the needs and feelings of others and to understand and resolve some of his own needs with help. 5. He needs to know how to accept children of either sex as friends and how to interact with them socially in a way that is comfortable for him and them.

Let's explore each of these goals a little more fully. Your child will believe his own worth and beauty as you unconditionally love and accept him. That means by your words, actions, and the way you look at him you are consistently saying and meaning that he is lovable and valuable. Even when you must punish him or are angry with him, you may honestly explain that the reason for such actions and feelings is that you care about what he becomes and how he acts. Furthermore, he will feel good about himself as he accomplishes tasks and learns to act in a way that makes you as parents proud of him. A compliment for picking up toys or playing quietly can create a glow of pride on a child's face. It is a major achievement for a preschooler to eat a meal without spilling anything. A phone call to a grandma, so a child may share such an achievement with her, will further enhance his sense of worth.

Self-acceptance will inevitably come to include the respect and appreciation of others. Your child's feelings toward others will clearly mirror yours as parents. If he constantly hears you criticizing or condemning him or another person, he will learn to be suspicious or disrespectful. But if you take the trouble to find out why someone acts in a seemingly rude or thoughtless way, and explain this to your child, he will learn to understand and feel compassion for others.

We have already discussed ways to help a child know the differences between the sexes. By your comments about men and women as sexual beings, your child will or will not learn to accept and value both maleness and femaleness as a whole.

It is by respecting a child's need for privacy and by teaching him to respect yours, that his respect for others increases. This has great usefulness in school, when children do their own work and are not constantly intruding in other students' activities. Children also learn respect when their ideas and interests are seen as important to their parents. When you as parents listen to your child and respond to him with warmth and concern, you are teaching him respect that will be of value to his whole life.

Children will accept both sexes naturally when they are not taught otherwise. It has come to be considered "cute" to tease very young children about having "boyfriends" or "girl friends." It always surprises me that five- and six-year-olds seem to understand this as having sexual implications. They will bristle in anger or they may laugh with those who tease, but they get the message that maybe they are supposed to start such relationships early. Childhood is very short at best, and it is sad to see it abbreviated even more by such teasing, with its implications. For many reasons, I would urge you to avoid such teasing and caution your family or relatives to respect this policy.

Social Aspects

The young child interacts almost exclusively with the parents and family and an occasional or regular baby-sitter. This fact is good in terms of providing the consistency babies need to form patterns of safety and trust in their human environment. As young children reach the age of three, however, they are ready to play and socialize with other children in active ways. Before they are three, they do play with each other, but it involves mainly independent play in the midst of others.

Children playing with other children, sometimes older ones, involves certain risks. To handle such risks, parents need to be near or provide adequate supervision of their children. Due to excessive curiosity from either too much, too little, or the wrong sort of sex education, many children will explore each other's bodies while at play. Some of this exploration is natural, but it can be both frightening and guilt producing to a child. Few parents are prepared to handle such a situation well. They may try to ignore it, think it's cute, or most often react in panic with lectures and punishing. A child is likely to respond negatively to these reactions.

The most meaningful solution is to gently draw aside the children who are involved and have a little chat. Explain to them that all children have a natural interest in their own bodies and a curiosity about other people's bodies. Tell them that to undress with each other, however, or to handle each others' bodies can feel scary and that it may give them upset feelings such as you probably see demonstrated on their faces. Suggest that they let you (or their own parents), explain to them from a book what they want to know and then help them get on with better play activities. Be careful not to teach more to someone else's child than they would want him to know.

Children can become sexually excited, and to become involved in experiences that create such intense feelings so prematurely may cut short the carefree simple joys they deserve. If a playmate of your child persists in such activities, try to discuss it with the child's parents. If they are unable to help, it may be necessary to keep that child away for a time. Most children do stop such behavior after a while.

Seeing parents involved in sexual intercourse is usually highly upsetting to a child. Although I know that many people, citing more primitive life-styles, disagree, in our Western culture at this time, I maintain that such behavior is inappropriate. Sexual intercourse is the most intimate and intense experience in family life. It allows no room for a third party. The child is excluded and may feel abandoned. Also the sounds and physical actions are certainly different from any familiar part of a child's life. This may frighten him. Often the child finds himself greatly excited and even sexually aroused and has no outlet for such feelings—except perhaps to experiment with a sibling or a child next door!

During my elementary-school years, I knew two six-year-olds, a boy and a girl, who would go alone into a small storage room near the play area at school. Being curious and wishing they would come and play with me, I peeked through the keyhole. To my uninformed amazement, they were engaged in sexual intercourse in an adult fashion. I now know that these children came from families where privacy was not a part of sex. It is not surprising to me that both of these children became sexually promiscuous in their teens.

There are many aspects of parenting that are not convenient! To have to postpone your own sexual pleasure may be frustrating. One answer may be to allow some scheduled time away for a second honeymoon, while grandparents enjoy the children. Another is to plan the children's sleep and activities so as to allow some privacy for yourselves. It is also possible to teach children to give you some time with each other while they play or watch TV. When you live in a small apartment and have no relatives close by, this problem becomes even more difficult. Sometimes friends will trade child care, or your own creative minds may think of answers. Certainly true lovers can find a way.

It is important to find a balance in the social attitudes and activities of your young child. On the one hand, he needs to feel unashamed and even proud of his body. He needs to be comfortable with physical affection between his parents and among friends and family. On the other hand, his awareness of adult, intense sexual activities needs to be postponed until he is older and is capable of understanding the complex interactions of all of the factors that are a part of a healthy sex life.

Spiritual Aspects

There are several spiritual lessons your preschooler may learn that relate to sexuality. God is a very orderly being. As I have learned how every living creature can be classified scientifically into a relatively simple array according to their complexity, I am in awe at God's genius. Little children, by learning that their physical design and differences have a meaning and a reason planned especially by God, the Creator, may get a glimpse of what God is like. By knowing that God put such planning and effort into creating people just right, they may also come to see their own personal value and develop the reverence for life that is seriously lacking in today's world.

Children, as I have experienced them, have a natural awareness and awe in spiritual realms. My grandson, at the age of two and a half, grows wide-eyed with wonder at a fuzzy caterpillar. His excitement over squirrels and birds reminds me that they, too, are a wonder. As children increase in their understanding of God's creation of male and female, perhaps they can really come to know that in His sight we are equal even if different. And maybe there will be hope that the battle of the sexes may end, and we can live together in peace and joy!

7
Time Out

While the preschool years are full of significant developments, sexual ones as well as others, during the elementary-school years other areas are of greater interest to children.

One worried mother came to me about her seven-year-old daughter. Polly was immensely concerned about boys. If her favored one of the month (or week) was not attentive enough, she would brood. When he failed to call her in the evening, she worried and even cried at times. She was a precocious child and had overheard her parents' arguments and struggles in their troubled marriage. She had apparently turned to a boyfriend, even at this tender age, for some sense of belonging and caring. She actually played out with him many of the conflicts and uncertainties of her parents' relationship.

Polly's story, however, is unusual. It is much more likely that parents will be bothered because Craig has blackened the eye of David in a fight over whose turn it was on the tire swing. Or Joyce is in tears because Sally played with Stephanie during recess instead of with her.

Physical Influences

Physically, growth of the grade-school child has slowed to a crawl. The only reason to buy new jeans in an entire season is that

Arnold has worn them threadbare climbing up and down to his tree house.

There is great emphasis on competition, and fights, especially among boys, are almost universal. Boys speak a competitive language. How he wrestles and how far he can jump is what concerns a boy, not what shade of color goes with this, and how he combs his hair. Appearance rarely concerns a boy. He seeks out other boys with whom he can compare himself. At a very elementary level he exchanges views on whether or not his muscles are like other boys', whether he can jump or play ball as well as other boys, and whether his penis is like other boys'. They handle each other —sometimes manually, sometimes through observation, and sometimes verbally.

This is not abnormal and need not worry parents unless a child becomes preoccupied. Sexual development is not a nice, gradual, measurable process. It takes place in spurts, just as the entire physical development of a child does. Boys need to belong to a group so they can compare and develop a sense of loyalty. Their willingness and ability to contribute some pleasure and strength to that group holds them together. As they compare themselves favorably in some regard, they learn later on to become separate, whole, independent human beings.

During a performance, a successful gospel singer spoke of feeling very inferior as a boy. He described himself as having pimples and loving to eat green onions so girls were, he felt, repelled by him. He said that unless you've experienced it, you don't know how it feels to have both team captains fighting over you—because neither of them wants you on his team! Many a boy who has not found a place in a group knows how that feels.

Teachers and parents need to be aware of the boy who lacks physical skills and feels inadequate. With help and practice, these skills can be developed at least enough to help each child fit into a team at some level. Learning to swim, skate, ski, and play tennis not only provides healthy recreation and respect from other children but also provides avenues for social activities in healthy dating relationships later.

Girls also compare themselves with each other. They are typically, however, more likely to compare hair length and style rather than muscle size and physical skills. Girls tend to seek an ally— a best friend—and rarely identify with a group unless an adult organizes it. They team up together against other girls and against their common enemy, the boy. While this is not always true, it generally tends to be so and this tendency needs to be modified by watchful parents. Exclusion of others allows for jealousy, cliquishness, and creates shaky foundations for adulthood.

While boys and girls need much time alone with friends of the same sex, boys and girls also need to play and work together. Getting to know members of the opposite sex as friends and competitors nonsexually, enables them to see each other later on as whole people and not just sex objects. In physical activities they can learn respect for each other as well as themselves.

Even within a family, a brother and sister can learn to love and respect each other. David and Kimberly fought as bitterly as most brothers and sisters do. But when Kim learned to run fast enough to beat David in a grade-school track meet, he buried the hatchet. He proudly told his mother, "She runs just like a boy!" Kim was no less a girl, but the skill she developed earned a place of respect for her as a person and helped stop some of the competition between her and her brother.

Physical Problems

Physical development is of great importance in establishing a child's self-image and his position with his friends. There are some physical symptoms that often show up in the elementary-school child that need to be discussed. One of these is excessive weight gain. There are physical causes of this that need to be checked out by a doctor, but usually this is a sign of emotional distress. Loneliness, boredom, and even anger may be temporarily forgotten in the enjoyment of food. In their worry about an overweight child, many parents resort to nagging or using threats such as, "The girls won't like you if you're fat!" Such an approach only intensifies the child's feelings, and he may feel compelled to eat all the more. He may even sneak or steal to get food. Instead of scolding, parents need to find out what is hurting the child and causing his emotional hunger. When his needs are satisfied and he feels safe and important, he usually will forget the desire for food.

Other physical problems common to elementary-level children are these: stomachaches, headaches, and sometimes aches in the legs or arms. These complaints, too, need good medical evaluations. Commonly, however, they are symptoms of personal problems or difficulties in school.

Lorie's parents brought her to me for an examination because she awoke every morning with a tightness in her stomach. She said it felt like a knot there, and she often felt too sick to go to school. She was surprised to remember that it didn't bother her on Saturday or Sunday. As we talked, she poured out this story: A boy sitting beside her had trouble with his lessons. He would often peek at her papers or ask her for answers. She didn't want to tattle on him or hurt his feelings, and she was afraid the teacher would find out and blame her for allowing him to cheat. She was in a double bind. It seemed there would be trouble whatever direction she took. To make matters even worse, Lorie liked the boy and didn't want to lose his friendship. With a little help from her mother, Lorie was able to ask that her seat be moved, and the stomachaches disappeared. Physical, emotional, and social factors are closely intertwined.

Another physical-sexual problem of childhood involves masturbation. Most parents become worried if they discover that their children handle their genital areas. During the childhood years, this is important if it becomes excessive or if it produces guilt.

Marilyn was sent to me by her teacher because she was preoccupied with her genital area. She would masturbate openly and at almost any time. The teacher's private suggestions and reminders that this made other children uncomfortable were to no avail. Marilyn lived in a family that was quite open about sexual matters, but they had little time for her. She was in a neighborhood where there were few other children, and she was very lonely. Somehow she had discovered that her major pleasure in life could come from her own body. The masturbation became a habit that she was unwilling to break. Through counseling, her parents came to understand Marilyn's emotional needs, and they were able to take the time to show her more love and to teach her to play with toys and friends, and to find pleasure in areas outside her own body. In a few weeks the masturbation had stopped.

When I was a child, I overheard my mother telling an older sister about a neighbor who had to be committed to a mental hospital. In a serious and worried voice she said, "They say it's because he masturbated so much!" Parents may deal with a child's masturbating in a way that produces intense guilt. Even overhearing this comment made me afraid of the end results of such an awful habit. Now we know it is unresolved fear and guilt that may produce serious mental problems, not masturbation itself. In this neighbor, as in the case of Marilyn, the masturbation was a symptom of his illness rather than the cause of it.

Sexual response is as normal as any part of life. When a child is forced through shame or fear to regard normal sexual response as sinful or harmful, it may become a problem.

At two, baby Andy had an erection of his little penis during a diaper change. His face lit up with the pleasurable feeling he experienced. His grandmother, instead of scolding him or hurrying to rediaper him, smiled back and said, "Andy that feels good, doesn't it? Isn't God wonderful to make our bodies so they can feel so nice?" Andy listened and I know he will forget the words. With repetition, however, I hope he remembers that we are "fearfully and wonderfully made" by our Creator (Psalms 139:14). Healthy adult sexuality is based on such attitudes.

There is another view of masturbation that is held by many sincere people. This position holds that all masturbation is wrong because it is a purely sensual pleasure. Since it is also a purely self-centered action, this point of view is a valid one.

In normal people, it is possible for sexual issues to become a preoccupation. When this happens, we need to take a look at our lives in their entirety. If our attention becomes focused on any one aspect of life to the exclusion of others, we are in danger of getting out of balance. Imbalance needs to be evaluated and corrected before it causes major difficulty.

A patient I once worked with kept herself in a state of constant anxiety over the issue of masturbation. She believed that it was a sin and yet she often was tempted to indulge in it. She was single and had no other avenue for sexual expression since her conscience forbade sexual intercourse even more intensely than masturbation. She was trapped between her physical needs and her conscience. When she indulged in masturbation, she would suffer from intense guilt. When she refrained, however, she would experience severe sexual frustration. It took a long time to resolve her dilemma.

This young woman decided that for her, masturbation was wrong, and she chose to refrain from practicing it. She learned to avoid sexually stimulating books or media presentations. She disciplined her thoughts to areas of life apart from sex. She consumed her energy in exercise and other creative activities. She invested her love in friendships with many people. For her, the indecision was a factor in causing anxiety. Once the choice was made, the energy she had wasted in her internal struggles could be used to find creative answers.

Emotional Influences

During the grade-school years, emotional forces are hard at work molding our children's lives. Fear is the cornerstone of adult sexual impotence or frigidity. And in the helplessness of childhood, fear can become deeply rooted. Anger is the source of the resentments we have seen that are such a barrier to the freedom and warmth of a good marriage. Love is the healing and protective emotion that must be carefully taught and consistently demonstrated for a child to believe it and learn to live by it.

Fear

Here is an example of the destructiveness of fear in one boy's life. Larry's father coached his baseball team and was himself a good player. Larry wanted more than anything in the world to play baseball in a way that would make his dad proud of him. He was not very well coordinated and his intense desire to do well made him panic. He would, so he recalled, look at his dad, the coach, for some sign of encouragement or pride. If it was ever there, Larry missed it. He sadly struggled through one miserable season of failure after another until he was old enough to quit. A really bright young man, Larry's fear of failure became so great that he dropped out of college and made a living as a cabdriver. Larry has never married and is afraid to risk a committed relationship. He is afraid that he can't measure up as a man, just as he failed to measure up in baseball as a boy.

Children's best mirrors of their worth are the eyes of their parents. When parents' eyes too often reflect scorn, disappointment, or indifference, the child will inevitably develop a self-image that matches.

Not only is parental pride and approval important to the growing child but so is that of his teacher. Next to the parents, a teacher may be the greatest human influence in a child's life. Frankie, at five, was short, shy, and the youngest child in kindergarten. When he was tired, he would occasionally revert to sucking his thumb, a habit that comforted him. His kindergarten teacher felt it was her duty to take from him this last stronghold of earlier dependent times and make him grow up. She stood this shy little boy in front of a roomful of twenty-two other children and required him to suck his thumb. She told these children to laugh at him. Frankie was crushed. Paradoxically, only the fact that this teacher was equally cruel to other children in his class saved some of his self-respect, but he was afraid of his teachers for many years.

Another teacher, by contrast, recognized that Sarah, at nine years, was a child who was extremely deprived and abused. She learned that Sarah had never owned a doll and bought one for her. Since Sarah's mother would not allow her to take it home, this kind teacher would require Sarah to stay after school to do some extra reading. As a reward for her efforts, Sarah and the teacher would then play with the doll. Through years of difficulty beyond belief, Sarah held on to the memory of that doll and the tenderness of the teacher who cared enough to stay late and play dolls with her. It was the only pattern she knew for mothering her own two children.

Parents need to be informed about a child's teacher. When abuse or neglect in a classroom tears down the confidence parents have worked so hard to build, a change is in order. Most teachers do care and if parents explain the needs of their child, a good solution can be worked out. If that isn't the case, however, you as parents may need to seek the help of a school counselor or principal to resolve such a problem.

Other children's ridicule and rejection are the last major fear of most children that we will discuss here. Teasing by a brother, sister, or playmate can be devastating. Many a failing child whom I have interviewed is preoccupied with name calling: "Fatty," "Skinny," "Dummy," "Long nose," "Buck teeth," or "Rooster tail" (for unruly hair), can contribute to a child's inferiority complex in life-defeating measure. Laughing at mistakes or differences may come from one child's discomfort, but ridicule may deal a deathblow to anyone's self-confidence.

Many grade-school children are so unsure of themselves that they simply can't deal with a child who is significantly different. They can, however, be taught and helped to do so. Parents need to be aware of such a situation and teach their children to understand and accept others who do not fit the usual pattern of child behavior. Parents need to teach ground rules for children's disagreements that prevent physical or personal attacks and hurt feelings. Teachers may be even more helpful at this point than parents. Allowing a child to experience his own pain, as part of life, is one way to help him empathize, or feel for, someone else's hurts. It is tempting to rescue or overprotect our children, but there are times when they need to feel pain. Parents and teachers can use such experiences to teach children to be compassionate and to care about someone else's heartaches.

One excellent and creative teacher of first graders decided to teach them how to show compassion, rather than ridicule, for problem children. She spent five or ten minutes each day telling a story that would illustrate such a value or having a child share an event that caused pain to him, such as losing a pet or a friend's moving away. These small children were invited to do or say anything they chose to help or comfort the hurting classmate.

They surprised the teacher by their ability to comfort and show compassion to someone in need.

Reaching out to help and encourage others can be taught just as readily as can teasing and ridiculing. What a lot of self-esteem and interpersonal warmth could be generated by this way of life. And what a warm, loving, sexual relationship could be the natural expression of such lives later on in a marriage!

Anger

A major problem in sexual adjustment, as we learned earlier, is that of anger. Whether it is the withholding of love by a passive, stubborn spouse, or the aggressive demands of a willful, controlling one, anger can create trouble. The habits we as adults use in expressing anger were formed in childhood. During school years, there are many opportunities to teach children to understand and use their anger in healthy, constructive ways.

An example of the result of failing to teach a child to use anger well is the story of Paula. She usually enjoyed sexual relations with her husband, Burt. But after their second child was born, Burt began to feel overburdened and worried about keeping up with the costs of supporting the family. His interest in sex declined and their personal relationship suffered. Furthermore, Burt insisted that Paula spend less money and demanded accountability from her regarding finances. Paula was angry and resistant, but Burt steadfastly held his ground. Paula refused to have sex with him and slept on the couch. In counseling, as we looked at her stubborn refusal to respond to the reality of Burt's logic, Paula revealed a habit that began in her childhood. When she wanted a favor from her father, she could usually make him give in by pouting and acting angry. When she realized how childish she was being, Paula gave up trying to always have her own way, and her loving relationship with Burt was restored.

Paula, as a child, needed to learn to work out disagreements by reasoning and logic instead of by manipulation through anger and tears. Had Paula's father known that he was allowing a habit to be set for life, he could have held firm when necessary and avoided giving in to her pouting.

Children can learn more readily than adults how to express their anger wisely. Here's how you may teach them—and yourself, if you need to know. First, identify and name the exact feeling: irritation, frustration, anger, fury, rage, or whatever you experience. Thinking of the name for it gives you more control over it and the emotion less control over you! Second, think about what it was that stirred up such a reaction in you or your child. Children usually are quick with this answer: "Janie took my cookie!" "Bobby broke my doll!" Finally, decide what you will do about the situation. Children aren't sure how much power they have to do anything. As a parent, you can help with, "Here's another cookie. Now eat it where Janie can't get to it." "Let's fix that doll and put it on your shelf so Bobby can't reach it."

Teaching children how to use what power they do have is an excellent beginning for internal, adult strength that is solid and real and doesn't have to be proved in destructive or manipulative ways.

A good feeling of love and warmth can so easily be encouraged in a child, and equally as easily destroyed. Alice, a teenager with severe problems, told this story. Her father had repeatedly scolded her for her poor grades. She worked hard to improve and excitedly ran home from school, eager to show her first good grade card to her dad. He was sitting in his easy chair watching television after a hard day's work. Alice handed him the card, eagerly awaiting his surprise and praise, but her heart turned to stone as he silently threw the still-folded card on the floor. He didn't even see it! That day Alice gave up. She decided that she would never again try to please her father. In fact, she felt that forever would not be long enough to get even with him through rebelling.

Even well-intentioned discipline may end up in serious emotional damage to a child. Carol's father, a minister, had high standards for his children. He was consistent in enforcing them, and his methods were successful—but emotionally deadly. He would take the culprit alone into his study and sternly explain what his crime had been. He would spank him and send him away. He carefully stayed coldly angry and thoroughly disapproving of the offending child for at least three days, just to make certain that he knew how bad he had been. To Carol that seemed an eternity. Her effusive personality could hardly wait to be restored to her father's good graces, and she always feared that he might never forgive her. As an adult, Carol had serious problems in her marriage, living in constant fear that her husband would repeat the rejection and cold anger she had grown to know in her father.

Love

It is relatively easy to love a child. The parent who awakens each child with a kiss instead of shouts will start a better day—and will be teaching the child how to be a loving person himself. Following necessary and fair discipline with forgiving and loving restoration will heal while it teaches. And consistency will cement the foundation of trust so essential in good relationships.

Finding time to tuck each child into bed at night is not just another expression of love. It is also a good time for confidences. Keeping good communications open, as we have discussed, is fundamental to good sex education. That type of communication begins in childhood. The vulnerability a child often feels at the end of the day can open up great conversations and opportunities to demonstrate an understanding and loving spirit. The way you as a parent feel toward your child is usually how he will feel about himself and others.

Intellectual Influences

Intellectually, the normal schoolchild is extremely busy and challenged. So much information is so freely available that there is a danger of children knowing too much too soon. Corrie ten Boom tells us, in *The Hiding Place,* that her father made it clear to her that like a heavy trunk, too big for her to carry, sophisticated sexual knowledge was beyond her ability to handle at an early age. She reported that it was a relief for her not to have to try to understand adult issues as a schoolgirl. It may be tempting for parents in our "liberated" era to talk too freely and allow too much freedom and experimenting by children who need a sexual "time-out."

On the other hand, it is foolish and dangerous to assume that children know little or nothing. A sixth-grade boy was telling explicit sexual stories to his friends and was fast becoming a nuisance, if not a threat, to the girls in school. His parents, called by the worried administrator, were irate. They were confident that their son knew nothing of sexual matters. They had carefully protected his innocence and often asked him questions to test his knowledge. He consistently led them to believe he knew nothing. Actually, he was spending much time after school with older boys on his block. To maintain some status with them he was making up variations of their stories and using them to gain attention. Not wanting his parents to know and stop his game, he had been able to pretend his ignorance convincingly. Now please don't go to the other extreme and become a nosy, suspicious parent! Just keep an open mind, an open communication system, and an awareness that your child needs both your trust and your protection.

Outside Information

Sex education in schools has been a controversial issue throughout the United States. Many see the need for young people to know about sexuality and sex. Others fear the liberal and permissive climate that schools can create. As I've said before, don't worry—your child has had the most important part of his sex education from you, his parents, before he starts school. But there is a need for you as a parent to find out what your child is being taught in all areas of his schooling. You will find that much of the Family Life Education Series, or its parallels, is excellent. You may even use the material to get into some great parent-child discussions yourselves. In these talks, you may be sure that your child is learning the values and information you want him to have. But be sure to meet with your child's teacher and discuss with her your concerns about your child's information. Many teachers have told me that only at rare intervals does any parent respond to their invitations to come and discuss sex-education issues. Most teachers share your concerns and will appreciate your input if you do not set up obstacles. But the best of teachers and schools are no substitute for you as parents deciding together what is important and finding ways to teach that to your child in the framework of your special family values and beliefs.

It is important to define sexual role descriptions for grade-school children. Schools cannot do that. Probably no one can do it as well as you for your own child. How should a woman talk, walk, dress, and act? And what, besides his anatomy, makes a man different from a woman? How you parents act will teach these roles to your child. If he can understand, respect, and love you (and he will if you understand, respect, and love him!), he will know how to act when he grows up. No longer can we rely on our communities to teach these roles to our children. There are too many voices with too much truth and error in each one to depend on.

Television, magazines, and friends are all ready to teach sexual lessons. You as a parent need to be responsible for gaining enough information to know what attitudes your children are picking up. Be sure that in the process of this discovery you do not react with shaming or scolding.

A mother of a cute eleven-year-old boy, a baseball player and tree climber, was shocked to discover an adult magazine in his dresser drawer. It was carefully tucked away under his socks and T-shirts. Margie took time to stop, think, and pray for wisdom. What she did worked and seemed right to me. That night, when she tucked him in bed, she told her son that she had found the magazine and that it was still there under his clothes. Then she said, "Bill, I know you are almost a young man and that you have a natural interest and curiosity about women and men. God made us all so amazingly, it's okay to wonder and be curious about the perfectness and beauty of the body. I just want you to feel free to ask questions of your dad and me. You don't have to find out about sex and life from magazines and kids in a way that may not be wholesome and right. So maybe you'll want to throw that magazine away, but please do it only if you agree that it's best." Bill told his mother he hadn't felt right about the pictures and knew he was being sneaky. They discussed for some time his new sexual feelings and the long time he had to explore them. He understood there wasn't a hurry and that his parents would be there to talk with and help him know what he needed as he grew up. This conversation opened Bill's mind to a growing awareness and trust. He began to see that sex is wholesome and normal. Scolding, lecturing, or shaming Bill could have made him more deceitful and would have created a rift between him and his parents when he needed them the most.

Giving your child enough of the right information, along with your attitude of open wholesomeness, will help him form healthy attitudes and a good sense of his own responsibility. A child develops this sense of responsibility, you will remember, not by parental authority but by being given limited choices and by having watchful protection against his making serious mistakes. One of parenthood's most difficult and most frightening tasks is the gradual letting go and allowing a child the freedom to choose. Sometimes the child must even be allowed to make a mistake in order to learn, since the willful child often can learn *only* from experience. And to let that mistake teach the needed lesson without saying, "I told you so!" is difficult indeed.

Willpower

One last point in the mental development of the grade-school child relates to the child's will. James Dobson has written so well about dealing with strong-willed children and adults. Many stubborn children are growing up who are ready to listen to any new friend if he sounds exciting. Kids skip school because a friend suggests it; they experiment with drugs because someone offers them; they become sexually involved because "everybody's doing it." These children substitute the will of their friends for the wisdom of their parents.

A strong will is a great asset if it is directed in the right ways. While some children seem to be born with such a will, others must learn willpower with the help of their parents. When I was nine, my mother and I agreed I would learn to do fine needlework. She directed my efforts to a small pillow top with easy but solid embroidery. At first it was fun. The fabric was clean and the yarn bright and beautifully blended. But after a few square inches were done, it became tedious. I went out to play, and after a while Mother called me back. Reluctantly, I did a few more lines. Then followed the most miserable summer of my life—and, I'm sure, of hers. I cried, pouted, spoiled the design, hid the fabric, and resisted in every way a bright child could think of. Through all the fighting, my mother never quit. She corrected my mistakes, found the fabric, and literally forced me to finish that job. Then she put a pillow in it with a pink lining and a ruffle. She gave it a place of honor on the sofa in the parlor and proudly told everyone who visited that Gracie had made that. Despite my guilt, I felt some pride, too.

Many years later, during my first year in medical school, I was to relive a similar experience. The glamour and excitement of being in one of those coveted slots in medical school tarnished quickly under the stress of the incredible discipline and heavy responsibility of becoming a doctor. I wanted more than anything to quit. But it was a worthwhile goal and I had learned long ago to finish a difficult job, because my mother cared enough to see to it that I learned to use my will correctly and not to quit.

It is this principle and its early enforcement by parents that will enable young people to develop appropriate values and find the strength to live by them. It must be taught early, when the child is young and adaptable enough for the parent to manage and to discipline, as did my tenacious mother. A few years later would have been too late.

Social Influences

Social skills during the elementary-school time are year by year forming patterns that will be used later in the dating period.

Self-esteem

Interpersonal relations depend almost totally on the individual's own self-esteem. While this has been mentioned often before, it needs to be reinforced. As the child sees himself, so he will tend to see others. Both school and home must cooperate to find and encourage success experiences. And these need to come from the expression and development of each child's unique gifts and talents.

Every child needs to look well. It needn't take much money, but the careful selection of colors and styles in clothes and haircuts can enhance the person's natural beauty. Giving the growing child some choice in shopping also increases his self-confidence and experience in decision making.

During the depression of the 1930s, I was in grade school. Often we could afford fabric for only one school dress, but shopping for that was an exciting event. The material was handled fondly and sewn carefully. Whenever a friend would drop in, Mother would insist I bring out that fabric or newly made dress and show it to the guest. She always said some variation of, "Isn't that nice material? Gracie always chooses something so dainty!" I remember feeling that it was I who was special, not the fabric. Life is made up of such extremely important little things!

In today's hurried world, people often forget the social significance of good manners. Compliments on and the noticing of little everyday courtesies can increase such good manners. Compliments need to be simple, to the point, and deeply honest. I can hear some parents say, "But my child never does anything well!" Every child does something well! In trying to be good parents, we tend to focus on our child's problems so we can correct them. Unfortunately, we take for granted the nice things that don't need correcting.

A friend was trying to change her habit of yelling at her children in constant disapproval and irritation. One hot summer day they repeatedly ran into the house from playing in the yard for drinks of water. Every child allowed the door to bang so loudly that the mother was fast losing her resolve to be kind. She asked the children each time they entered to please close the door quietly. At last, as she neared her breaking point, one child remembered to hold the door to prevent its bang. My friend gave that child a quiet but grateful hug and a special "Thank you!" It wasn't long before the others were carefully silencing that door so that they, too, could be praised and hugged. Courtesy, kindness, and encouragement are so important in a child's security and self-esteem, and they carry over in all of his social relationships, as well.

Parental Assistance

Not only does each child need self-esteen but he also needs to respect and like other children—both boys and girls. Social comfort with children of the opposite sex depends on training and life experiences. But a major influence is that of the parent of the opposite sex. As children see their parents get along with each other, they realize that both men and women are safe and loving. As they experience the love and esteem of both parents, they feel valued. But as a boy senses his mother's approval and love, he will learn to return that and transfer it to other women and girls. And as a girl feels her dad's admiration and protection, she will learn to trust other men and boys who are like him.

This special attention from the parent of the opposite sex needs to be balanced with the necessary discipline and common sense. If only one parent is in charge of discipline, there will be some complicated problems. Mark was his mother's favorite. His father was gone much of the time, and his mother depended on his moral support and love for her strength. She rarely denied his wishes and never punished his mischievous ways. In adolescence, Mark became involved in drug abuse, sexual relations that resulted in the pregnancy of a teenage girl friend, and in general, was ruining his life and wasting a fine mind. Being loving and proud of a child does not mean being permissive or blind to misbehavior.

Knowing how to get along happily with boys and girls may call for parental assistance. Recently I worked with a third-grade boy who was lonely and socially very different from the other children. His parents were strict and did not allow television in their home. Don was at a complete loss when the other children talked about "Mr. Rogers' Neighborhood" or reruns of "Gilligan's Island." He withdrew into a world of spaceships and monsters. I felt especially sad for Don because I could remember my own childhood. Not having a radio, I felt totally left out when the kids laughed at "Fibber McGee and Molly" or mimicked "Digger O'Dell." By no means are television and radio the only areas of sharing, but children must have some common interests in order to communicate meaningfully.

Sports and games, teachers and school, parents and neighbors are also interests children share. Helping them to converse at home by listening and responding to their ideas and experiences will teach children that they have something worth saying. Obviously, children can and must learn to listen, as well. The child who is allowed to be too much the center of a family may become the nonstop talker who bores his friends and estranges every date later on.

It is most helpful to encourage your children's friends to be in your yard or home at least part of the time. This enables you to see what your child's strengths and weaknesses are in his social adjustment. It gives you an opportunity to know and guide his choice of friends and may even enable you to influence these friends in some positive ways. A few broken windows or drinking glasses are a cheap price for these benefits.

As a Camp Fire Girls leader and Cub Scout den mother, I had a wealth of experience with groups of young boys and girls. When a boy walked by while the girls were on a hike, it was common to hear a chorus of "Oh! Cooties!" I felt sorry for the boy, so scathingly put down, until a comparable group of boys, seeing a girl, would moan in unison, "Oh! Cooties!" While I know much of this is in fun and some is a protection against the confusion and uncertainty of the soon-to-come world of boy-girl relations, some is just plain meanness. In today's world, with its battle of the sexes, perhaps we need to discourage such disparagement. I believe boys and girls can like and respect each other and need not hurt anyone's feelings.

Spiritual Influences

Spiritually, grade schoolers are still teachable. The biblical precepts of kindness, compassion, and love are what we've been talking about. Both the Jewish and Christian beliefs portray the godly life as desirable and one that relies for guidance and strength on a transcending power. When children are fortunate enough to have parents who exemplify this loving, guiding power, it makes it much easier for the child to transfer trust to the heavenly Father. As parents teach obedience to their child, he finds it possible to obey the laws of God.

As a child learns increasingly complex facts of science and math, and experiences the creativity of literature, art, and music, he can learn a proportionately growing awareness and reverence for God, the ultimate Wisdom and Creator. Learning the amazing order and perfection of the atom and how its layers of electrons and protons resemble our own solar system is again convincing of a Master Mind that is essential to an orderly universe. The infinite variation of the universe from microscopic to the macrocosm surely includes concern for individual and unique persons. Parents and the church need to join forces to keep accurate information before the child to remind him of the logic as well as the revelation of a God who cares, is ultimately powerful, who is looking after his total good, and who is wise and strong enough to set him free to choose. Finally, it is prayer that may influence that choice aright.

Childhood evidences so graciously the qualities of forgiving, understanding, learning, and growing. The persistent "Why?" and "How?" challenge us all as adults. It's no wonder Jesus said, "Except you become as little children, you can't even enter the kingdom of heaven" (*see* Matthew 18:3).

8

Almost There: Adolescence

Adolescence is like building a second story on a house. Its security
depends on a strong foundation being laid in early childhood and
a solid first story being built during the grade-school years. It will
be essential, therefore, to review what your adolescent learned
during his earlier years. Now don't panic and throw up your hands
in despair if your earlier building job was faulty! It's not too late
to go back and make repairs. It's more difficult and takes some time
and energy, but it's so important that you do it! Be sure that you
understand what you have been reading.

Physical Aspects of Puberty

Since physical adolescence, or puberty, is taking place earlier
than a generation ago, you need to be aware that this chapter
applies to the preadolescent child as well as the teenager. Across
the country we are hearing of and seeing girls as young as ten or
eleven becoming pregnant. On the other hand, there are many
young people who show no signs that they are developing sexually until their midteens. When to teach the concepts in this chapter, then, depends on your watchful, sensitive awareness of your
particular child's readiness. If you should err, let it be on the side
of too much too soon rather than too little too late.

Very few biological factors cause more profound physical
changes than does puberty. The glands throughout the body that

stimulate growth and promote health operate with incredible efficiency by an individualized time clock. We know that heredity
and general well-being affect the ticking of the clock, but just
what triggers the alarm ring of the onset of puberty, no one knows.

The levels of the special secretions called hormones have been
building silently and gradually, causing small bodily changes for
several years before the major changes of early adolescence take
place.

The master regulators of this complicated process are the hypothalamus (part of the brain) and the pituitary gland. They are
located in the skull, carefully protected by a bony case, and attached to the base of the brain. The chemicals they send out go
to the testicles or male sex glands that are in the scrotum or sac
at the base of the penis, and to the ovaries or female sex glands
located within the pelvis of girls (*see* picture). In the testes and
ovaries, these chemicals stimulate the production of the primary
sex hormones of estrogen (female hormone) and testosterone
(male hormone). It is most important for you to understand that
all girls and women have a little testosterone (mainly from the
adrenal glands) and a lot of estrogen while males have a little
estrogen and mostly testosterone. Hormones from the thyroid and
adrenal glands also add to the process of sexual development.

Estrogen causes the development of breast tissue in both boys
and girls. In my pediatric practice, I saw many twelve- and thirteen-year-old boys who were alarmed because of swelling under
the nipples. They feared cancer or some mysterious illness or were
sure they were doomed to be "sissies"! After checking to be sure
nothing was seriously wrong, I could confidently reassure them
that this swelling was normal and as soon as the testosterone
secretion increased in their bodies, it would disappear. Studies
have shown, by the way, that hormones do not cause homosexuality.

Female Puberty

Estrogen in girls brings about many more changes than in boys.
It stimulates the continuing growth of breasts to the full size each
girl's genes and chromosomes planned for her to have. It is unfor-

tunate that today's Western society has equated sexual desirability and even femininity with large breasts. Many flat-chested girls suffer real mental anguish because they believe they compare unfavorably with other girls. The small-breasted woman is just as lovely, just as feminine, and just as able to nurse her children as those who are more generously endowed. Teenagers need to be reassured and taught to accept themselves just as they are, physically as well as in all other ways. If they have learned the self-esteem we've been considering up to now, you can see how much easier it is to add the acceptance of their physical appearance as a teenager.

In the ovaries and the uterus, estrogen interacts with several other hormones to cause ovulation and menstruation. Ovulation is the process in which a microscopic egg (ovum) which has lain sleeping in the ovary begins to grow and is pushed out of its tiny pocket into the body cavity in the pelvis. Normally it is sucked up at once by the soft, waving motions of the fimbria into one of the Fallopian tubes, then moved gently into the womb (*see* picture).

While the ovary has been busy producing the ovum, the womb has been at work building up a velvety lining, rich with little blood vessels and nourishing fluid. If the egg is united with a sperm while it is in the Fallopian tube or the womb, it will rest on this soft uterine lining and then nestle in to begin the long process of becoming a baby. If it is not fertilized by the male sperm, it will die in a day or two and later will pass out of the womb along with some blood, serum, and tissue that were waiting for it. This is called menstruation. Many years ago, I was told, a medical student described this process as "the weeping of a disappointed womb." While this is picturesque language for the womb, it doesn't always describe the feeling of the woman!

The process of ovulation takes place about once every four weeks. Usually this happens midway between menstrual periods, though it may be as early as one week after or as late as a week before the period. While the average menstrual cycle is twenty-eight days, many women have shorter or longer ones. The period of menstruation may last from three days or less to a week or more. Not only do these facts vary from woman to woman but occasionally within a person, as well. This does not necessarily mean there is anything wrong.

A change in schedule, moving, emotional upsets, physical ill-nesses, and many other factors may influence the delicate and intricate processes that are responsible for women's menstrual periods. Furthermore, it may take many months, or even years, for a young woman to settle into her individual cycle. It is important to know this to avoid worry and to realize the importance of being sexually responsible. Many girls believe that ovulation does not take place in the early months of their menstrual periods. While ovulation is irregular at first, it does frequently occur from the very first period, and as soon as ovulation begins, pregnancy can take place. I have seen several pregnant young girls who did not know this significant fact!

The signs of trouble with a girl's menstruation need to be noted. For these, a physician should be consulted. 1. A total irregularity of periods continuing two years after menarche (the first period). 2. Excessive bleeding—using more than one regular box of pads or tampons (and soaking them) per period. 3. Bleeding between regu-lar periods. 4. Severe pain, cramping, and especially a tendency to faint during a period. Usually these symptoms do not indicate serious trouble, but a physical evaluation by a competent doctor can reassure both the girl and her parents.

Every girl needs to understand menstruation and be prepared for it before it takes place. You need to watch your daughter for signs of her sexual development. The growth of hair in the pubic area (groin) and under the arms usually begins about one year before menstruation will take place. The growth of breast tissue also precedes this process by one or two years. While it may be difficult to see these changes in girls, who prefer a great deal of privacy, your awareness will help. Don't be afraid to ask your daughter, and by all means, as soon as you even suspect that she is approaching puberty, discuss it with her and tell her what to expect.

Because you, the mother, or an older daughter began menstrua-tion at age fourteen is no reason to believe any other girls in your family will also start at that age. Each woman has her own special alarm clock. So observe, think, and talk. Tell your daughter what is beginning to happen to her, what it means, and how to take care of herself physically as well as socially. The possibility of pregnancy needs to be explained, and at this time, I believe it is urgently important that each girl learn about sexual intercourse and pregnancy.

As a young adolescent, I did not know how a girl became pregnant. I knew only that a missed menstrual period might mean pregnancy. So when I was late (and I was one of those irregular people) I would worry. Perhaps, I feared, I had become pregnant from a toilet seat or the abhorred kisses of my girl friend's overly affectionate father. In my reserved family, I did not know that I could have asked and found reassurance. Unnecessary worry could so easily have been prevented had I been taught the simple facts about sexual relations and conception.

Debbie, at twelve, was pregnant and in a home for unwed mothers. The social worker, in taking a history, asked her when she had started to date. Debbie looked at her in utter amazement. "Why, Mrs. Jones," she said, "I'm too young to date!" Debbie tragically taught me that sex education needs to be a constant process and that rules are not enough. She had become pregnant while on a walk during halftime at a basketball game.

An almost universal problem related to menstrual periods is the physical pain that accompanies them. In Genesis, we are told that as a result of Eve's disobedience to God's orders against eating the fruit of the tree of knowledge of good and evil, she would have to bear her young in sorrow and pain. Today, a slang expression for menstruation is "the curse." Many girls exaggerate this discomfort and some even take advantage of it to gain an extra day in bed, but there is no doubt that it is an uncomfortable and even miserable time for some.

As part of the hormone cycle that is responsible for menstrual periods, for a week or more before their periods women store up fluid in their bodies' tissues. This may amount to several pounds and will, in most women, produce a feeling of physical heaviness and emotional tension. They cry easily, feel gloomy, have headaches and a tendency to be explosively angry. Unfortunately, many women today deny this process because they feel it means they are in some way inferior to men. Instead of denying them, women need to be aware of these physical differences in order to take good care of their bodies.

Besides the fluid accumulation, there are other factors that cause menstrual cramps or discomfort. One of these is the increased size of blood vessels in the pelvic area. Sometimes constipation may add to the sense of pelvic pressure. General fatigue or mild infections such as colds or flu are likely to affect the degree of discomfort.

There is a remarkable influence on menstrual discomfort by one's attitude. Carol began her menstruation at the age of eleven. She resented the inconvenience of those monthly periods and felt especially put upon since none of her friends as yet shared in this experience. She was irritable and moody and struggled against the discomfort, needing a heating pad, several hours in bed, and constant sympathy. After some months of such general misery, she said to her mother, "Well, I guess there's not a thing in the world I can do about it, so I'll just have to make the best of it." She put away the heating pad, initiated daily exercises, ate a balanced diet, and tried to get extra rest during the more difficult days. Carol's attitude didn't eliminate all the discomfort, but it enabled her to cope successfully with the realities of life and helped her develop maturity and wisdom.

A relatively new discovery shows that severe menstrual cramps are associated with the level of still another hormonelike substance called "prostaglandin." While this discovery is new and the treatment is experimental, there is great promise of real relief from the few truly severe cases of menstrual misery caused by this.

The use of pads and tampons to absorb the menstrual flow is historic. For several decades, schools have shown films and led discussions for preadolescent girls and their mothers. These are wonderful opportunities for parents to teach, guide, and share in this important event in their daughters' lives. A mother's sharing of the memories and feelings of her own puberty can draw her daughter close in a bond of understanding. This is the time for a mother to invite her child into the world of womanhood and begin teaching her how to become a beautiful woman. By accepting the fact of her daughter's new, though incomplete, adulthood many of the troublesome mother-daughter conflicts of the teen years can be avoided.

Finally, the use of tampons needs to be discussed. The wide-spread mass-media advertising campaigns leave little privacy to today's woman, so various sanitary supplies are well known. Tampons are specially made devices that fit into the vagina and absorb the menstrual flow directly from the womb. They are convenient, comfortable, and allow more freedom than do pads in activities such as swimming. Some people believe, however, that they cannot be used by a young woman who is a virgin.

Let me explain that in girls there is a protective membrane that partially covers the opening to the vagina. It is called the "hymen" and protects a child from getting dirt or germs into the genital area. Normally, there is an opening in this that adequately allows for the flow of the menstrual discharge and is usually big enough to easily insert a tampon. Some mothers have found their daughters using these without their knowledge and panic, thinking the girl has had sexual intercourse and broken the hymen. This is not necessarily true. It is possible for the hymen to tear through strenuous activities or minor injuries. On the other hand, in less than 10 percent of women, the hymen is so tough and the opening so small that tampons cannot be used. Such young women may need to consult a physician regarding possible treatment for this condition.

Newspapers have widely publicized a rare but occasionally fatal disease called "toxic shock syndrome," which may occur during menstruation. Gynecologists believe the evidence relating this syndrome to the use of tampons is as yet inconclusive. It would be wise for each woman to consult her doctor on this subject.

Boys also need to understand the process of menstruation in girls. The proper time to discuss it is not as crucial as with girls, but they may avoid or better handle some embarrassing situations by knowing about this process before they start dating. Occasionally a girl will have an accident while menstruating, resulting in blood stains on her clothing. If boys understand this, they need not stare or laugh out of their uneasiness. When a boy starts dating, there will be some times when his special girl simply doesn't feel like taking part in a tennis game or going swimming. If the boy understands why, he can help her choose a quieter event or simply postpone the date without embarrassment.

Many young people today discuss sexual issues of all sorts very openly, and much of this seems wholesome. When a girl's period, however, is called "the curse" or she is described as being "on the rag," I feel the negative implication is far from wholesome! A simple explanation by a girl that she is having her period seems quite acceptable. If a girl is not comfortable even with this, how-ever, the boy who knows can value her privacy and not press her for explanations.

I see no reason that a boy should not be told the entire story about ovulation and menstruation, just as a girl is told. He needs, however, to hear it in the framework of respect and dignity, not uneasiness, ridicule, or put-downs. The use of proper words rather than slang is a part of both good attitudes and right information. Please refer to the list of definitions for the most common terms and their meanings.

Testosterone in girls, like estrogen in boys, is present but not dramatic in its effect. It causes some deepening of the voice and some hair growth in the underarm and groin areas and on the legs. Girls are as different in the kind and amount of hair growth as in breast size. Often it is limited to the areas above, but it may include hairs on the chin, chest, arms, and around the nipples. While our society portrays this as ugly and unfeminine, it is quite normal. Most young women prefer to shave their body hair or use a cream (depilatory) to remove it. There is a process called "elec-trolysis" that can permanently remove unsightly hair. Parents need to understand how embarrassing it is to an adolescent to be very different from her friends and help her to take care of this part of puberty.

Unusually coarse or thick body or facial hair on a girl may be due to a serious physical problem, such as a tumor. Be sure to consult a physician if you or your daughter are worried. At any rate, an annual physical examination is a good habit to teach your child.

Male Puberty

Now let's turn our focus to puberty in boys. Testosterone in boys produces dramatic changes, also, though they are very different from those caused by estrogen in girls. As the male hormone, along with hormones from the pituitary gland, build their concentration in boys, they begin to grow rapidly. To support this growth spurt, the body requires food, and during this time, boys' stomachs become bottomless pits. As their arms and legs grow long, they feel and are awkward and uncomfortable. Hair begins to grow over their bodies and usually is longer and coarser than that on girls. Their lips become fuller and hair starts growing on their faces. The larynx or Adam's apple grows and their voices become octaves lower. Early in the process of this change of voice, it may slip in the course of one word from a childish soprano to a deep bass, causing great embarrassment to a boy. The testes and penis slowly enlarge to the adult size, and sexual feelings are experienced with a new impact.

As important as are all the physical changes that are taking place in a young man at puberty, the most significant happening is the production of sperm cells. In response to the stimulation of the hormone testosterone, a boy's testicles start making the cells that, when united with the female egg (ovum), begin a new life. These amazing half-cells contain in their microscopic size everything except nutrients that are needed to make a perfect baby with fingers and toes, a brain, heart, and every part of a body. The color of skin, hair, and eyes, of course, will vary, depending on the genetic makeup of the parents.

Seminal fluid, in which sperm cells swim about, is being made in the prostate gland and seminal vesicles (*see* picture). During sexual intercourse, this fluid, loaded with millions of sperm cells, is discharged forcefully in the female's vagina and uterus or womb. The sperm move quickly to the ovum if it is present in the womb, but only one of all the millions will reach and fertilize it. The other sperm will die and be discharged from the vagina. During intercourse, a little muscular valve will close the opening from the urinary bladder to the penis so the urine does not damage the sperm cells.

The temperature required for the development of healthy sperm is 2.2° C lower than the temperature inside the body. The location of the testicles outside the body in the scrotum maintains precisely the required temperature. Occasionally, a young boy may have one or both testicles in the abdomen rather than in his scrotum. This condition, called an "undescended testicle," needs to be checked periodically by a physician. Usually at puberty or before, the testicle will come through a natural opening into the scrotum. If it does not, a doctor may need to perform a simple surgical procedure to put it in place. Unless the testicle is in its proper place, it cannot produce sperm and the man will be sterile, or unable to help conceive a child.

While boys have nothing like the monthly menstrual period of girls, they do experience something that can cause them alarm. At the time boys are developing sperm and are getting ready for adult sexual functioning, they begin to have "nocturnal emissions." This is a fancy medical term for a "wet dream." Boys commonly have dreams of a sexual nature, and as part of those dreams, the penis becomes erect and an ejaculation takes place. Sometimes they recall the dream; other times they do not. Young men may fear they have wet the bed and may be embarrassed and afraid. Or they may feel that they are immoral and struggle with guilt. Parents need to explain that this is perfectly normal. It is the body's way of releasing sexual tension and of preparing for sexual intercourse later in marriage.

Not only boys but many men, as well, are tortured by guilt feelings about nocturnal emissions. They feel that their dreams are evidence of the sin of lust on their part. To such men I would like to give reassurance and hope. The nocturnal emission, far from being an evidence of guilt, is God's plan for your release from sexual tension.

It is common for adolescent boys to compare their physical characteristics with each other, just as girls do. The boy who is shorter, less muscular, has less body hair, and a smaller penis may be thrown into despair. Unfortunately, group showers after gym classes make it impossible for adolescents to maintain any privacy. The girl who hardly needs a 32 A bra may be driven to a major inferiority complex by her friend's 34 C! These feelings, illogical as they are, are nonetheless real and tragically painful to the adolescent.

Parents need to teach and reassure their adolescents that: 1. Physical development is slower and later in some than in others and this is a time to be patient. 2. Personal worth is the product of who we are inside and completely transcends stature and genital size. This is a time to explore and develop those qualities of being that will make all of life more delightful. 3. Respect for and sensitivity to the feelings and needs of other young people is much more useful than physical competition and comparison.

It is in communicating these personal values to their adolescents that parents need to be aware of their own sexual attitudes and ideas. In order for children to believe their parents, how the parents act must be in keeping with what they say. Several adolescent patients of mine reflect confusion when their parents behave in a flirtatious or seductive way with friends, while telling their teenagers not to act that way.

Just as girls fear that they may be sexually and socially undesirable to boys, so do young men fear that they may not be appealing to girls. Many boys worry about performing sexually when the time comes for marriage. Learning that sexual relations are a natural physiological process, as are nocturnal emissions and all of the other biological functions, can help a boy to relax and wait for the right person and time for this. God created people as sexual beings, and if we do not interfere through wrong attitudes and mistaken information, sexual functioning, with all of its marvelous meanings, will develop unmarred in our maturing children.

Masturbation

Masturbation, ever present and always an area for confusion and guilt, may take place during adolescence, just as it did in childhood. During these years, however, it often takes on almost a quality of desperation. As young people occasionally experience an adult sexual orgasm during masturbation, they may become preoccupied with repeating this exciting experience. Since a sexual orgasm involves complex physical, emotional, and mental interaction, it may not always be achieved easily. The young person then fears that he or she is abnormal, or perhaps through guilt, may believe God is punishing them by taking away their sexuality.

Parents need to talk about masturbation with their teenagers. You may explain something like this: "Sally [or Jim], I've been wanting to talk with you a bit about an issue I know many young people are concerned with. It is masturbation. I want you to know that almost everyone may do this at some time or another. It feels good and the fantasies one often has during this are exciting and stimulating. It's comforting to know that you are a normal, sexual girl [or boy].

"Becoming too involved in masturbating, however, can use up a lot of your time and energy. If occasionally you awaken from a dream sexually frustrated, or for some other reason you do masturbate, realize that the guilt feelings that result are natural. You may find yourself thinking about sex so much that your mind is not free for school and other activities. You can easily translate feelings into thoughts, thoughts into fantasies, and those fantasies into more intense feelings, until a vicious cycle develops that is hard to get out of.

"If you find yourself in such a vicious cycle, please come and talk with us. We can help you find ways to stop this and turn your attention and energy to other interests and activities.

"Sexual experiences are so special that you should save them for marriage. Masturbating may release your tension and help you control those powerful sexual drives, but remember that the God who created you will guide you and help you control yourself and your relationships and keep them right and wholesome.

"Once you are married, of course, this problem will evaporate. Then the normal, loving relationship you and your husband [wife] have will be meaningfully expressed in intercourse with each other. I once knew a couple who expressed their anger toward each other by refusing to have sexual relations. They would masturbate instead, and finally their marriage broke up. I hope you'll never be so childish, but will find an exciting, fulfilling relationship in every way in your future marriage."

In talking about sexual matters with your children, be as relaxed as you can. Ask them questions. Pause at times for a point to be well heard or a question to be asked. If you are comfortable, your child will be relaxed, too. So talk over these matters with each other as mother and father or with a reliable friend, if you are a single parent, until you are at ease.

Hygiene

Puberty brings with it the need for special attention to personal hygiene. There is an increase in oil and sweat secretion by skin glands after puberty. The hair becomes oily, and there will be an offensive odor unless the young person bathes frequently and learns to use a deodorant. Deodorants of many names and types contain a chemical that decreases perspiration in a local area, slows down the growth of skin bacteria, and allows a pleasant rather than a sour body odor.

Boys often believe it is "sissy" to use a deodorant and think it is manly to neglect cleanliness. Many rebellious young people have avoided bathing and skin care in general. Fortunately this neglect seems to be subsiding, and we see more and more clean and well-groomed young people.

A major problem of teenagers is a condition in which red bumps with a white point appear on the skin, especially over the face and back. These may turn yellowish and become ugly pustules which are often painful. Some people are more troubled with these than others. Girls are especially likely to have a crop of them before their menstrual periods. This condition is commonly called "acne," and may require the care of a dermatologist, or skin specialist.

The following rules, however, will help many boys and girls keep their skin quite clear: 1. Avoid a diet of too many fatty foods or sweets. Cola drinks, chocolate, fried foods, or rich foods should be greatly limited. Eat plenty of fresh fruits, vegetables, and a moderate amount of meat and eggs. Drink plenty of water. 2. Keep the skin clean and soft. Wash thoroughly morning and night with a gentle soap, dry carefully, apply a small amount of lotion to soften the skin and keep the pores open at night. In the morning the use of an astringent to close the pores and keep out bacteria will help prevent infections of the sweat and oil glands. A common astringent is denatured or "rubbing" alcohol. 3. When there is a tendency for the skin to become infected, an antibiotic may need to be ordered by a doctor. Antibiotic ointments are available without prescriptions and may be used on each pustule to prevent the spread of the bacteria when these break. 4. It is important to avoid picking or squeezing these spots to prevent more serious infections or even blood poisoning. 5. Acne is often more prominent on the forehead and along the hairline, so it is very important to keep the hair clean and prevent oily secretions that accumulate in the hair from adding to those of the skin. 6. Remember that this condition is almost always limited to adolescence, and the day will surely come when the youth will outgrow it!

Sexual Curiosity

Ours is a world that is preoccupied with sex. Recently someone quoted a television programmer as saying, "If we don't include some sex in our programs every five minutes, we believe we'll lose our audience." Besides television, one has only to look at magazine and paperback book racks to see blatant and often vulgar sex advertised to all readers.

Many viewers are curious young people, and they are often stimulated by what they see, to the point of wanting to go and try it for themselves. These young people may even begin their dating with a plan to get to the point of sexual intercourse as soon as possible in order to experience the excitement and pleasure that is implied by what they see and hear. This is sad, because the intensity of the sexual activity is great, and it may crowd out a great many other worthwhile experiences a couple needs to explore.

Polly, a high-school senior, once came to me for advice because she was pregnant. She and her fiancé had been having sexual relations for some months but felt they were not ready for marriage. It was their decision that she have an abortion, and together they went through this painful experience. Fortunately neither of them took this lightly, and experienced great heartache over the loss of what would have been their first child. Later they decided to resist having sexual relations until they were married. Polly told me that their relationship only began to develop at that point. They discovered interests and activities they will share all of their lives. Previously, they had been so involved sexually that they simply had not enough time and energy to explore the broader and deeper aspects of life.

Whether a young couple plan to get to intercourse quickly or their relationship simply evolves to that, it is important for boys and girls who are dating to know the natural biological progression that takes place in "petting" or "making out." Usually this starts with hand holding, walking arm-in-arm, and perhaps a good-night hug and kiss. Depending on the values and viewpoint of the couple, however, the physical relationship may progress quickly or more slowly to long periods of kissing, embracing, and touching or caressing of each other's bodies. At some time in this sequence, one or both may reach a point of no return, when the urge to complete sexual intercourse becomes almost uncontrollable. In fact, if there is not a release of the semen by the boy, he may become intensely uncomfortable physically, and the girl may be equally frustrated emotionally.

Each person needs to assume the responsibility not only for himself but also for the other person, so their relationship does not reach this point until they are ready for marriage. A girl needs to understand that she can arouse a boy's sexual feelings by the way she acts and dresses. A boy needs to realize that girls, too, have intense sexual feelings. To tease and play to the point of this sexual intensity and then suddenly cut off the interaction is pain-fully frustrating. To allow the progression to end in intercourse is risky at best and may totally spoil a relationship.

I know it sounds old-fashioned to make a plea for abstinence (not having sexual intercourse) before marriage. But so many physical as well as emotional and social problems are involved that I believe every couple should avoid premarital intercourse. The possibility of an untimely pregnancy, even in today's world of contraception (prevention of pregnancy), is only one risk. Confusion regarding a series of sexual partners may make one feel cheap and often sexual promiscuity (intercourse with many different partners) is merely an exploitation of one by the other. Such selfishness inevitably results in one or both persons involved being hurt.

Emotional Aspects of Puberty

You can see what a complex, finely tuned mechanism is the physical aspect of sexual functioning. Emotionally, we are just as intricate! Confusion, fear, and responsibility of growing up are all made painfully clear to the adolescent through the physical processes. But how can he or she cope with these emotions?

Kathy began her menstrual periods at age thirteen. She was intellectually prepared for menarche but went off to school the next day with considerable apprehension. Her mother, understanding the significance of this momentous occasion, picked her up after school that day rather than having her ride the bus, as she usually did. As Kathy got into the car she groaned, "Oh, Mother, this has been the worst day of my life!" Her mother replied, "I'm sorry you were so uncomfortable! Why didn't you go to the nurse for some aspirin?" Then followed a most revealing comment. "It wasn't the physical pain, Mom. I feel fine. It's just the first time in my life something has happened to me that I can't do a thing about!"

Kathy had lost an era of time: the carefree playtime of childhood was gone. It would never return, and she had, without a decision or even a vote, been moved into the world of young womanhood. The frustration and even anger that Kathy expressed was a part of a normal process of grief over her loss. Her mother understood this and tried to help her through this "passageway" into an exciting and fulfilling new era of time. Some parents do not understand, and their children must grope their own way through.

Grief, anger, and helplessness, as displayed by Kathy's story, are only part of the emotional upheaval of puberty. There are, for many young people, serious fears. These fears are shared by both boys and girls and relate to the following issues:

First, teenagers fear unfavorable physical comparison with their friends. This has been explained above, but briefly, teenagers fear looking very different, being too fat, too buxom, too tall or short, too fat or thin.

Second, adolescents fear that they will not be socially acceptable as young adults. This fear is especially real for those who have not had close friends or who lack self-confidence. Girls who wait for boys to call them for a date have agonizing visions of a lifetime of spinsterhood spent by a silent telephone! Boys, in turn, may sit frozen by their own telephones dreading the imagined despair of a turndown by that special girl.

Third, not only do adolescents fear their physical and social inadequacies but they also fear a more intangible, poorly defined specter of not "making it" sexually. The "macho" and "sexpot" images so touted by society today can be intimidating to the best of adults. Small wonder, then, that measuring up must seem so impossible to youth.

A recent movie, *Looking for Mr. Goodbar,* dramatically exemplifies this fear. A young homosexual man, in a frantic attempt to achieve sexual relations with a girl, goes crazy and kills the girl in a wild outburst of fear and anger with himself. The very depiction of such an event reveals that tragically, such feelings do occur in our world, where sex has become a goal or an ideal rather than a normal biological function. Sex was designed by God to happen naturally and beautifully, when husband and wife are ready. It is not a way of proving manhood or womanliness.

In a desperate attempt to prove themselves, many young people make up stories of sexual feats. One sixth-grade boy told tales of getting his girl friend to undress with him. However, he told the story to a group in which, unknown to him, was the older brother of this girl. A fight ensued in which the braggart was roundly beaten by the brother. This sort of boasting may be harmless in most cases, but very often it leads to fantasies of an ever-increasing sort that sooner or later will be acted out in real sexual exploits. When sexual acts are based on efforts to prove oneself instead of expressing mature, unselfish love, they will bring heartache and disappointment rather than fulfillment and joy.

As parents, it is your responsibility to explain strong emotions to your adolescents. Helping them understand that they are not alone or different can be most reassuring. You may find your own way to tell them but here are some suggestions:

An appropriate story from your own memory bank can draw you close to one another through understanding. Be careful to avoid stories that might give subtle permission to irresponsible behavior.

Discuss episodes shown on television. These are plentiful and show every nuance of sex from very good and responsible to highly immoral and destructive. This requires thought and critical analysis, but it can open some profitable conversations that may teach important concepts. Avoid being drawn into angry arguments, however, that can cut off communication rather than opening it.

Keep your eyes and ears open to events and articles that can illustrate a principle. Be aware that lectures and moralizing are usually wasted on teenagers! Whatever you say, keep it short, conversational, and factual. Your young adults have their own minds now, and they will interpret for themselves the truths you give them. At this time in their lives, you need to trust all your previous good work as parents. It will pay off well now.

When young people talk about their feelings, a marvelous thing happens—especially when they have a good listener. As they talk, the intensity of their emotions is drained off. Solutions to needs and problems begin to seem possible. A plan of action can then take shape. But best of all, the unconscious need to act out feelings in ways that can be dangerous disappears. So listen, respond, share, and *care,* parents. That's one way to teach your adolescent about the emotional aspects of sex.

9

Other Aspects of Adolescence

The impact of puberty on the life of a child is immense. The physical and emotional aspects of this have been discussed. Every adult, however, needs no book to recall his own adolescence with its contrasts and frustrations. As you remember, therefore, let's think together about the interpersonal or social arena in which these inner conflicts are struggled through.

Social Aspects of Adolescence

Family Relationships

Let's begin this discussion with the interactions of the family. In chapter twelve we will talk about the need for the preschool child to spend constructive time with the parent of the opposite sex with the approval of the parent of the same sex. That same rule applies in the years of adolescence. Boys need to know their mothers and to enjoy thinking, working, and playing with them in order to know how to relate to their wives later on. And their dads need not feel crowded out or resentful. Obviously, dads and sons must continue to spend their own time together in order to set the patterns for manhood which the boy also needs. And to complete the picture, there must be time together as a whole family to offer role models for man-woman, husband-wife, father-mother, and whole person. Reverse the pronouns and you can see that a girl needs time with her father, and so forth.

Several years ago, a woman named Laura called me, deeply worried about her youngest daughter. Julie had been a hardworking child in school and helpful at home. She enjoyed her friends, took part in sports, and was active in her youth group at church. At thirteen, however, Julie was starting to notice boys and wanted to begin dating. Laura felt that Julie was too young and lacked the sense of responsibility so important in this part of her life.

The problem was not, however, with Julie. In Laura's opinion, it was with Julie's father. From birth, Julie had been the "apple of his eye." She could do no wrong, according to her father, and she knew precisely how to stay in his good graces. Laura had often worried about her husband's spoiling their daughter, but saw her good qualities and reasoned away her fears. Now, with the serious responsibilities of young womanhood facing her, Laura could no longer wish away her worries.

Visiting with both parents together, we discovered an all-too-common situation. To some degree, in fact, it is almost universal. As the parent of the opposite sex becomes a little (or sometimes a lot!) too lenient, the other parent gradually becomes more critical, and even harsh. This imbalance may increase to the point of an open and explosive conflict. There is a psychiatric name for this called the Oedipus Complex (for boys) or the Electra Complex (for girls).

While this conflict is usually mild and often can be handled by a session or two with a counselor, sometimes it becomes so violent that it may be damaging to the whole family. When Laura's husband, Paul, understood her concerns, he could see that he had overlooked too many issues and had left the limit setting to his wife. As he began to take part in setting up rules and disciplines, Laura gratefully relaxed and could enjoy her daughter. Julie learned to respect her dad more as he stopped giving in to her manipulations. The vague sense of guilt Julie had felt when she sensed her parents' disagreement over her disappeared. Waiting to date became easier for her as her family life became harmonious.

Contrast with this example the following disguised but true-life situation. Debbie's mother was in emotional pain because her husband always took their daughter's side in a controversy. Pat felt—and indeed was—powerless, even in situations where Debbie's safety was compromised by her father's decisions. They refused to accept counsel and instead isolated themselves—Dad in his study, Mother in her bedroom, and Debbie with her boyfriend. Debbie acted out her needs and confusion by becoming sexually involved with him. Only when she became pregnant did this family find help.

Within the family, problems often arise out of the extremes in interpersonal relations. When parents overreact, children may be pushed to rebel. One bright, attractive, unwed mother I worked with related her mother's overprotectiveness. This mother required her daughter, a college student, to account for every minute of time and to relate in detail every activity in which she took part. Her mother's constant demands for an accounting of her daughter's behavior pushed the young woman too far. She said, "I finally had to get pregnant to prove to my mother she couldn't control everything I did!" A high price to pay for overreaction and rebellion!

Indifference or not caring enough to set limits for young people is the opposite extreme to overreacting. This has produced its share of problems, too. More times than I care to count, I have heard troubled young people say, "My parents let me get by with anything! I don't think they even care about me." Such teens keep testing the limits, to see if their parents care enough to take a stand. Tragic indeed is the family where that caring is missing or is so inconsistent that young people must keep testing it out through disobedience or risky behavior.

Parents who discipline their adolescents through shaming them or making threats are also asking for trouble. Disciplining by making a child feel guilty is a certain means of destroying that essential quality of self-esteem. Making such remarks as, "If you don't stop going out with Don, you'll end up just like your Aunt Elsie!" (who bore an illegitimate child), can produce exactly the disaster the parent fears. We call this a self-fulfilling prophecy. One young lady I counseled during the course of her unwed pregnancy said, "My dad called me a tramp so often when I didn't deserve it that I decided to get even. I've got the name anyway, so I'll just play the game!" A number of people suffered for that double mistake.

Other Relationships

Outside the family, young people need to be taught how to relate comfortably with the opposite sex. In any relationship, people go through at least five stages. First, there is the ritual of meeting and greeting a new person. Second is the small talk or pastimes by which we gradually get to know one another's way of life. The third stage involves sharing activities and exploring each other's interests and skills. Fourth is the ability to be apart from each other and still maintain the friendship. Fifth is the stage of intimacy (not sexual) in which we can reveal deep feelings of any sort, in a trusting fashion, without hurting or being hurt by each other. In any relationship, one may stop at the stage that is most comfortable. While most people do well to reach stage three with a few priceless friends, we may move on to true intimacy. The family sets the pattern for all social relationships. As parents and children learn to be honest and trusting in their interactions, children will learn to relate comfortably with others outside the home.

Young people who have a variety of activities and skills to share and develop rarely have problems socially or with sexual preoccupation. They are so busy learning and doing that they just haven't time for adult sexual activities. It is instead the lonely youth, afraid of his own image, who seeks to prove himself or find the warmth of some affection, who is vulnerable to premature sexual relationships. Or it is the teenager who covers insecurity with a pretense of sophistication who may search for sexual excitement.

Sherrie, a college junior, came to me for counsel during an unplanned pregnancy. Her parents were alcoholics who showed much emotion but little real love. When Sherrie went away to college, she was so lonely that she moved in with a young man. She said, "The lovemaking was okay, I guess, though I wasn't too crazy about that. What I did like was waking up every morning with someone's arm around me!" She learned, sadly, that even a man's arms around her did not constitute real love. As soon as he knew she was pregnant, he left.

The mother of a thirteen-year-old girl recently found her daughter in the process of undressing with her eighth-grade boyfriend. This girl was one who had been taught good values and seemed to have plenty of friends and success experiences. As she and her mother talked later, she said, "Mother, in our crowd almost everyone has had sex. I simply can't be the only one who is a prude!" Her mother gently explained the painful consequences of early sexual experimentation, and a real crisis was avoided. Going along with the crowd is so important to adolescents. It takes great wisdom and courage for both parents and child to dare to be different!

Counteracting Adolescent Problems

In summary, these are the essential ingredients of social problems of adolescents that are likely to find sexual expression: 1. Competition or power struggles that may be fought through sexual issues. 2. Acting out of rebelliousness against parental strictness. 3. Testing the limits of parental inconsistency or seeming indifference. 4. Loneliness and a sense of inferiority that reach out at any cost for friendship or affection. 5. Joining the crowd or the "everybody's doing it" routine.

In order to help your teenager counteract these problems, here are some helpful suggestions. Some of them apply to you parents as well as they do to your children. When they do, you will find that your most convincing teaching is your consistent example in following them.

Feel so good about yourself that you can't help but feel good toward others. That means knowing and cultivating all the gifts, interests, and talents God gave you until you can enjoy them. It means facing squarely all the weaknesses and failures you have, working on those you need to change, and accepting those you can't change.

Choose to be a loving person and discipline yourself to act in loving ways. Love may be tough, demanding the best from the one who is loved, as well as tender, supporting a weakness in that person. But love is never rude or impatient. It is never selfish or ego centered. It does not sit back and wait for the other person to do something wrong and then find fault. Its toughness is gentle and kind.

Explore relationships with all kinds of people, using the five steps above, until you find the special people who best fit your interests, values, and with whom you become the best person possible. Out of those few, hopefully you will find the one you will want to marry. But don't be in a hurry. You need only one spouse!

Be affectionate and warm with all people according to your and their mutual comfort, but reserve sexual intimacy for the one special person you choose to marry.

As you seek to grow and improve yourself, be sensitive to all those about you, helping them in any way possible to become better people, just as you are becoming a better person.

While you are not ultimately responsible for others' needs or feelings, as your "brother's keeper" you are to be sensitive and responsive to him. Being loving means helping a friend in any way possible, and never exploiting or taking advantage of him.

Intellectual Aspects of Adolescence

Teenagers have so much to learn by experience and by listening. The physical changes alone are profound. After looking at the emotional and social issues they face, we can see that the problems of these years may seem gigantic to a young person. But the intellectual growth and maturation of an adolescent is a truly frightening process to many parents. We will limit this discussion to issues directly related to their sexuality.

1. Be sure your teen knows and understands the physical changes that go on in his own body and that of the opposite sex.

2. Especially make sure that your son or daughter understands the complicated interaction of sexual thoughts and fantasies with physical, sexual feelings in himself as well as in a person of the

opposite sex. This means he understands that sexual feelings stimulate ideas about sexual activity. These ideas lead to sexual fantasies or daydreams which stimulate more feelings, thoughts, and fantasies. The ever-increasing intensity of this progression may well lead to the acting out of those thoughts and fantasies. Many times the result is a tragic event that entails great heartache for everyone involved.

3. Be sure your child is responsible enough to control his own feelings, thoughts, and actions and to refrain from unfair teasing or seduction of a boy or girl friend—to protect himself and the other person from unnecessary risks. Knowing he can come to you, his parents, to talk about these feelings will almost always prevent his acting them out.

4. Values in all aspects of life are in need of clarification and strengthening during the teens. This is especially true in interpersonal and sexual areas.

5. Help your child to realistically accept himself and to love himself as his neighbor by accepting and loving him, yourself.

6. Require and help your child to make wise choices in every area of life. As he is capable, give him more of this responsibility and take less of it yourselves.

7. Remember and teach that wise choices must be based on logic and honesty, not desire or rationalization. It is very tempting to make a wish seem right even though we know it is not right.

8. Teach your child to develop his willpower. One may know very clearly what is right and wrong, but he may be so weak willed and poorly disciplined that he can't act on the information.

9. Teach your child to know God and understand His Word.

If you have made mistakes, parents, please be comforted! You are in a large crowd! Just consider yourselves blessed to know what the mistakes are, for then you can set about to correct them. Many people do not know or admit their errors and, therefore, can do nothing about them.

To be sure, we have all made mistakes, but don't forget that you have done many right things, as well. We may be grateful for and confident in these. We must trust our good parenting, the fertile minds of our children, and the care of our heavenly Father, and expect the best! It is tempting to make a last desperate effort in the teen years to redo all of our parenting. I have seen parents set up battles by lecturing, punishing, pleading, and threatening a child over temporary issues that could have gone by without incident. Overreacting is just as damaging as underestimating a problem.

A friend of mine relates this story about her only child, a son. She and his father had loved him dearly, disciplined him consistently, and had seen him become a fine young man. When he was in his late teens they nearly panicked for the first time. He began to date a girl with a very doubtful reputation. "In fact," said my friend, "it wasn't doubtful; it was simply gone!" The parents were anxious and perplexed. If they tried to stop him, he was old enough to rebel, and could quickly be lost to their love. They decided to trust their good parenting and his good judgment, and said nothing. In a few months, he had stopped dating this girl and had found a new and lovely girl whom he later married. Many years later my friend talked with her son about her concerns during that time. He looked at her in amazement and said, "Mother, I knew you and Dad always expected the best from me. I wouldn't have let you down for the world! I just needed to try to help that girl, because she really had some good in her." Whether or not that was the reason, their positive expectations paid off!

In order to be consistent with my philosophy of finding a balance in life, I need to remind you parents to keep your minds open to the worst as well as expecting the best. That may sound like a contradiction, but it really is loving "circumspectly," or by seeing the whole picture.

Shirley was fifteen and struggling. She was bright, restless, and had a hard time staying out of mischief. Her parents were proud of her and loved her deeply, but they couldn't always be sure of her good judgment. While they expected the best, they couldn't help but feel concern at times. A letter carelessly left open and available, perhaps in an unspoken request for help, revealed a relationship with a man that could have brought immense heartache to their child. By reading that letter, these parents were able to provide the protection this impulsive girl needed, and helped her avoid that pain. Watchfulness without accusations, prying, or lecturing is the key to the protectiveness of good parenting skills.

Spiritual Aspects of Adolescence

Spiritually, the adolescent is in a position to confirm or deny what he has previously been taught. His concept of God is fairly well set by now. It is true that most people unconsciously feel toward God as they do toward their fathers. Perhaps this is due to the prayer we were taught by Jesus: "Our Father which art in heaven . . ." (Matthew 6:9), or perhaps God, the Creator, made us so that we, as little children, could grasp the image of the heavenly Father through the loving care of an earthly father.

Certainly most of my own father's life and our relationship made it easy for me to love and trust in God. One day, however, a friend in a prayer group I attended asked me, "Why don't you ever ask God for anything for yourself?" Her question startled me, but I could not immediately answer her. Later, as I pondered this, a memory vividly returned to my mind. As a child, I had loved school. After the long, hot summers away from friends, I was always eager to get back to the times of playing—and even to studying—together. By early August, I would count the days until school started, and plague my busy father to take us to buy our new schoolbooks and supplies. My childhood was spent during the worst of the depression, and one year was particularly hard. My father valued education above everything except faith in God, but that year he kept putting off buying those school supplies. Only later did I discover that he had not wanted to worry us about the lack of money and that he had to borrow the few dollars it took to buy our books. By the time I discovered this, I had learned how much it worried my dad to borrow money. And because I appreciated his sacrifice for us, I vowed that I would never again ask him for anything that was not absolutely necessary.

I was totally unaware that I had transferred to my heavenly Father this loving concern for my dad. My heavenly Father is rich and able to give me whatever I need. As I realized that, a measure of faith I'd never explored before was released to me.

Teenagers just emerging from childhood are especially likely to look at God as being like Dad. For some that means God is permissive and rescuing and that His commandments may be nice but not particularly meaningful. For others God is rigid, unbending, and waiting to "lower the boom." Many young people rebel against this image of God, just as they rebel against their dads. To an increasing number of young people, God just isn't there, as Dad isn't.

It is of the utmost importance then, dads, for you to be available, consistent, protective, and caring—but not perfect. Your children will not expect you to *be* God, just the best you can be! You may make it easier or more difficult for your family to understand and trust in God. Today there are numerous families without fathers. Many parents have failed miserably. Let me repeat, "Do not despair!" Forgiving and changing are a part of growing! As parents forgive each other and themselves, they teach understanding and acceptance to their children. And God's love, forgiveness, and acceptance will be even more believable by the changes you and He make in your own lives.

In summary, these are the ideas young people need to grasp in order to affirm their own personal relationship with the heavenly Father.

1. God is not necessarily like Dad (though Dad may be a bit like Him!). He is loving, wise, and powerful. He punishes us only when He knows this is needed for our personal growth and improvement.

2. God's laws that specifically forbid adultery (sexual relations with another's husband or wife) and fornication (sexual relations before marriage) are for our protection and not merely to spoil our pleasure.

3. Submitting oneself to God does not take away from one's selfhood and is not limiting, except of evil and harm. Rather it is freeing and empowering to an infinite degree in positive, creative, loving ways of life.

4. Through Jesus Christ there is forgiving, healing, and power for overcoming all the sins and mistakes of one's life. Once forgiven, they are never remembered by Him again. (If only we

would be so good to ourselves!)

5. To a degree, it is possible to know God through the Bible, His followers, and the wisdom of His Holy Spirit. Through knowing Him, the understanding and love of oneself and others becomes possible, making us whole persons and enabling us to have healthy, exuberant, interpersonal relations.

6. God will never make you into a puppet. You always keep your power of choice. When you choose to love Him, yourself, and others, He will never leave you, but will stay by you to supply all your needs.

As you parents live by this knowledge, and as you help your teens to learn these facts, you can safely let go of them. They will, in His care and grace, be safe, truly free, and complete.

10

Concepts You Need to Know

There are several issues that closely relate to how to teach your child about sex, and yet they are controversial. I feel that you as parents need to understand and consider these issues.

Sexual Abuse

In my work with severely troubled children, adolescents, and adults, I have been amazed at the frequency of sexual abuse of children. In a survey of nearly eight hundred college students in the East, 19 percent of the women and 9 percent of the men reported at least one experience of sexual molestation during their childhood. Another authority estimates that if such a study included more people of different ages, those rates might be doubled. In many cases, this involves brothers and sisters, and less commonly, a father or stepfather. Uncles, grandfathers, and cousins round out a list that rarely includes a mother.

Commonly, incest (sexual relations between near relatives) is perpetrated upon girls, though there are cases where boys are the victims. Usually there are threats of revenge if the victim reveals the act, but often the child becomes frightened or angry and does tell. There is an amazingly frequent tendency for the mother to deny that such a thing could happen, and she may even blame the child for being seductive and causing it, if indeed she admits that it did take place.

In families where children see adults engaging in sexual intercourse, they may crave the physical closeness or become sexually aroused by seeing this intimacy. Often such children imitate this act with each other or other neighborhood children. Brothers and sisters, however, more commonly become sexually involved out of curiosity. There may be a power struggle between them that is expressed through sexual aggression. A boy who feels inadequate may believe he is powerful when he can force his sister to submit to his advances.

By no means is this problem of incest limited to deprived families. Incest is a common topic in letters to advice columnists and in articles in popular periodicals. It occurs in all levels of society and is so common that some sociologists are beginning to believe it is normal and should be ignored.

One father, however, caught in a web of his own making, found his daughter using their relationship to threaten him and gain her own way. It was he who finally admitted the problem and got help to stop it.

The problems with incest are many, but these are most common: A child instinctively fears, yet is sexually stimulated by, the sexual act with an older relative. Family roles and relationships become distorted and confused. This is especially true when a girl's father angrily threatens her one minute, then becomes "loving" and intensely physical, the next. His fear of her revealing the situation gives her an unwieldy power over him, on one hand. On the other hand, she knows she probably will submit to him again. The guilt, fear, and resentment that the child feels because the other parent tolerates this, adds further to her emotional burden.

Usually there is only one child in a family who is subjected to this treatment, and there may be a rivalry that ensues. Although the victim usually feels dirty and inferior, sometimes she may believe she is the favored one. One teenage girl knew both of her sisters had sexual relations with their father. She came to believe that she was ugly and undesirable because he did not approach her. This girl stated that she felt such sexual activity within her family was quite all right. Unfortunately, many people are beginning to agree with her.

The risk of becoming pregnant by a relative is always present. And out of such pregnancies, the chance of having a child with birth defects is greatly increased because of genetic factors. In close relatives, genes for some defect that would not show up if the other parent were unrelated are quite likely to coincide, causing that defect to materialize in their offspring. That accounts for the law forbidding siblings and first cousins to marry.

Men who initiate incestuous relations have several characteristics in common. They often are heavy drinkers, and drink to bolster their self-confidence. Almost always, they feel incompetent and childish themselves, and can't achieve an adult sexual relationship on a consistent level. They often are married to women who tend to take charge of the family, and they see that wife as domineering, frightening, and rejecting. Out of unconscious needs and feelings, they turn to their own children for love and support. When they demand submission from the children, such men may feel strong. This power temporarily meets those deep needs, and this drives the man to repeat the act again and again.

Perhaps such men, unable to find an emotionally satisfying relationship with their mothers or their wives, turn to their children for this. Since children also are incapable of satisfying this emotional need, all that may be left to the man is the physical relation. He can feel powerful and manly only relative to the helplessness of a child.

Girls who have suffered incest often become so sexually aroused that they later become sexually promiscuous in an unconscious effort to satisfy their deep and confused craving for love and protection. They suffer fear and guilt—but they also are angry and hurt.

It is not unusual for an angry, rebellious girl to falsely accuse her father of rape. At times, a girl's feelings for her dad may lead her to fantasize some sort of sexual experience and she may even dream about such an occurrence and come to believe it happened. Great sensitivity is necessary in evaluating such families and finding workable solutions to their problems.

Most authorities in this country agree that incest is seriously damaging to both child and family. It can be prevented by healthy sexual attitudes, information, and responsibility. If it's too late for prevention, good psychiatry and God's superhuman power and love can offer the solution.

Abortion

Another issue that is hotly contested in many magazines and newspapers is that of abortion. People are militant on both sides of this and a stance of logic and reason is hard to find or keep. Such noted conservatives as Dr. C. Everett Koop and Francis A. Schaeffer have offered superb insights to this question in *Whatever Happened to the Human Race?* But equally devout believers and profound thinkers have written another view in *Abortion: The Personal Dilemma* by R. F. Gardner.

I can add to the views of these wise people only personal, but I hope significant, pinpoints of insight.

The sight and smell of carnations will forever remind me of an untimely death. A beautiful young woman, my cousin, lay in a coffin banked with these lovely flowers. But they could not disguise the fact that she, who so loved life and laughter, was dead. She had been ill only a few days, and I, then a child, really did not know why she died. In hushed tones and guarded language, I overheard the grown-ups talk of "peritonitis" and her delirious ravings about her "sins." Much later I knew she had become pregnant and in an effort to rid herself of the disgrace so unbearable to her family, she had obtained an illegal abortion; an infection had set in and in a day without antibiotics, this girl had died.

Many years later, perhaps because of the indelible memory of such a wasted life, I became a director of a maternity home, a shelter for girls who became pregnant and bore children outside of marriage. In those days, it was still generally considered a disgrace to conceive and bear a child illegitimately. Over nine hundred such young women crossed the threshold of the home while I was there. I shared as deeply as one can in the heartaches and grief of those girls and their families. I felt there had to be an answer to their pain.

Then came the great era of freedom. State after state passed laws legalizing abortion. This seemed to be an answer to the pain of unplanned and unwanted pregnancies. There was no longer a need for twelve- and thirteen-year-old children to become pathetically premature mothers. They could go back to their dolls and record albums!

After some time, however, I began to be consulted by a pitiful parade of girls needing help. They had had abortions; sometimes more than one. They were full of remorse for their irresponsible taking of a human life—unborn, to be sure, but a life nevertheless. Many of these girls had serious issues of guilt and depression to resolve. But most did resolve them, put their lives back together with well-learned lessons, and grew.

I am more than a little troubled by seeing young people who admit to no feelings at all about an abortion. They claim to experience no remorse, no guilt, and not even curiosity about who that fetus might have become. I see young girls bent on habits of sexual activity that catapult them into a sophisticated and exciting lifestyle. Such a way of life, however, quickly turns them into hardened, tough people who seem to have lost the soft gentleness so linked with femininity in my memories and values.

When faced with an individual predicament, I am mentally tempted to join Dr. Gardner, who makes recommendations based on each situation. But philosophically and biblically, I join Koop and Schaeffer and say that if one must choose the least of ills, surely it is to choose life and not play God in its interruption.

Of all the painful components of an unplanned pregnancy, it seems to me the saddest is for a woman to choose and to go through an abortion alone. Many girls are abandoned by their lovers and afraid of the judgment of parents and friends. They are so alone and untrusting that they see no alternatives. Parents need to create a communication system with their children that encourages them to share their sins and failures as well as their successes. It is often out of such failure that we make our greatest growth in life, and wise parents may help turn problems into strength.

It is in the wake of sharing such tragic experiences that I gratefully remember the story in chapter eight of the Gospel of John. Ancient Jewish laws decreed that a woman caught in the act of adultery was to be stoned. A crowd of angry Jews brought just such a woman to Jesus in order to test His faithfulness to their laws.

With matchless wisdom, Jesus told them, "Let him who is without sin, throw the first stone." He refused to look at them, but bent down and wrote in the dirt. Silence grew as, one by one, all of the woman's accusers left her alone with Jesus. Surely His eyes must have twinkled as He looked at her and asked, "Where are your accusers? Is there no one left to condemn you?" Softly the woman answered, "Not one, Lord." Jesus' classic reply could only have redeemed the woman. He said, gently but firmly, "Neither do I condemn you. Go, and sin no more" (*see* John 8:3–11). An encounter with Jesus Christ can transform a life. His example is worth following.

Sexual Promiscuity

Many people would rather have their own way and rebel against the biblical injunctions against sex outside of marriage. Current studies are revealing medical problems that we cannot yet fully explain that are connected with sexual promiscuity. For example, cancer of the cervix is more common among women who have a variety of sexual partners. Venereal diseases, which we will discuss later in this chapter, are another obvious and serious risk.

While the physical risks of sexual promiscuity are easily evaluated, the emotional damage done by being sexually promiscuous is not so well understood. Let me relate some of the problems I have personally encountered in working with patients who have been sexually involved with many people.

There is a false belief that one's worth is verified by having people of the opposite sex attracted to him. In other words, one is acceptable if he or she is "sexy." This belief is historic but it has been cultivated by the movie and television industries today. Either knowingly or unconsciously, many people seem to have accepted this idea.

Usually subconsciously, many people feel that when they have been hurt or slighted enough by their spouse, this entitles them, guilt free, to retaliate by having an outside affair. Unfortunately, getting even does not solve the problem of the original hurt; it only complicates it and prevents the resolution and healing of that problem.

Avoidance of loneliness or boredom can be found through sexual relationships. One counselor has been quoted to me by his clients as having said to older married couples, "What you need is a new and stimulating relationship!" Unfortunately, for several people this resulted in divorce. The fallacy here is that happiness and fulfillment in life come from new relationships, and not from within ourselves.

An attempt to prove femininity, masculinity, and sexual desirability by a series of sexual partners is common among younger and older people alike. This seems to work at the time, but by the very fact of its repetition, it is evident that such proof is not lasting.

In our youth-conscious culture, there is a pathetic attempt, perhaps subconsciously, to regain one's lost youth through a young sexual partner. This device is at least as old as the great King David. In his extreme old age, he made a vain attempt to rejuvenate himself through beautiful young women (1 Kings 1:1–5). This did not help him. For many older men in our society, there is, temporarily at least, a sense of rejuvenation, but one can never regain lost youth.

The common denominator to all of these problems lies in the use of sexual encounters to try to prove something that either is not true or is not believed to be true. A search for solutions through a false premise is doomed to failure, and the end is even worse than the beginning. The many unwed mothers with whom I worked were prime examples. Not only did they fail to prove their beauty, find love, or achieve a permanent relationship with a man but they also ended up rejected, abandoned, and felt even worse about themselves and life.

Waiting for sexual fulfillment until marriage is not just an old-fashioned idea. It is a logical decision and sets a foundation through a choice based on broad areas of sharing life, and is not limited to physical attraction alone.

It takes courage and strength to make that commitment "for

better for worse, for richer for poorer, in sickness and in health, as long as we both shall live." Strength of character can grow only as it is exercised, and living out that commitment certainly provides the exercise.

In chapter five, we discussed sexual responsibility. I hope you can see, even more clearly now, how important that is. As you parents choose your private life-style, I hope the choice will not be based on what you can get by with, but on what is right and will make you a better, stronger person. Then you will be able to show as well as teach your children the reasons for their being sexually responsible.

Rape

Rape needs to be discussed because it happens so often and is such a violent invasion of one's personal rights. Rape is the forceful, violent act of sexual intercourse with an unwilling partner. Usually there are threats of harm or death unless the victim submits. Rape, reported and unreported, occurs somewhere almost every day. A number of months ago, a judge was roundly condemned for blaming rape on the seductive dress and behavior of women. While such behavior may be detrimental to a person, certainly rape is not caused by women. In fact, it is often committed on helpless, elderly women, or presexual girls.

The person who commits rape is a basically angry man who feels unusually worthless. When he is angry, this kind of man can become more easily sexually aroused to the point of sexual orgasm (or climax). The rapist, either unconsciously or by effort, allows his anger to mount until it becomes a force almost beyond his control. By acting out this anger through sexual aggression, he can feel powerful for a time, and is lifted out of his inadequacy. Usually this is a recurring pattern. Often, even after imprisonment, many such people are still a danger to society. The degree of violence varies from an almost gentle persistence to extreme violence that may cause the rapist to kill the victim and grossly mutilate the body. If every boy were loved and taught respect for himself and others, if he were helped to become successful and self-confident, there would be no rape. But as long as boys are humiliated, abused, and painfully neglected, we can expect retaliation in the form of rape.

As in the case of incest, there may be false accusations of rape. A young woman whom I counseled had become sexually involved with a neighborhood boy who was considered a rough character. The girl became pregnant and panicked at the thought of her parents' anger. She knew her parents would believe her if she accused the boy of rape. They did, as did the courts, and the young man was sent to prison for five years. However, as the date approached that the girl's child was to be born, her apprehension grew. Finally, she confessed the true story. The young man knew she was an innocent girl and had avoided her for a long time. It was her own craving for the attention of a man whom she saw as strong and protective that finally pushed her into seducing him. Even the best of judgments may be wrong!

Venereal Disease

The last topic we need to discuss that relates to the risks of sexual promiscuity is venereal disease. Since VD (the abbreviation for venereal disease) is reportedly at epidemic proportions in this country, let us briefly discuss the main types. Knowing about these will enable you to teach your teenager about the dangers of these diseases when they are unrecognized or untreated.

Gonorrhea

The most common form of VD is gonorrhea. It is caused by a germ that can be easily identified under an ordinary microscope. In the female cervix and vagina, this germ may live without causing much discomfort, though it often causes severe infection and great pain. During sexual intercourse with a woman who is infected with this germ, it is almost certain to infect the man's urethra and penis. This infection causes severe pain upon urination and a thick, yellowish discharge. The condition will, in time, tend to improve, but meanwhile he will infect anyone with whom he has sexual contact. Each, in turn, will infect other sexual contacts, and an epidemic is underway.

Though this germ is developing a resistance to the antibiotics that can kill it, gonorrhea is still quite easily cured by proper medical care. When untreated, however, it may cause such inflammation and scarring of the sensitive tissues in the reproductive tract, that sterility may result. A person so damaged may never be able to have children. A baby born to a mother who carries this germ in her vagina during its delivery is very likely to develop a serious eye infection. It is obvious that, when untreated, this disease has extremely serious complications that can be completely avoided by good medical care.

Venereal Warts

Another common form of VD is known as venereal warts. This disease causes the growth of wartlike tissue that is ugly and annoying, though not painful. The warts grow in a coarse, grayish brown cluster about the penis or on the labia. They are caused by a virus and must be treated by a physician, but they are entirely curable.

Syphilis

The most serious type of VD, because of its long-range complications, is syphilis. It is caused by a corkscrew shaped microscopic germ called a "spirochete." When this germ enters a human body through a scratch or even an irritated area of mucous membrane in the reproductive tract or elsewhere, it will cause a sore. This sore is only slightly painful, and for this reason, it may be dismissed as not being serious enough to require medical care. It heals very slowly, and is round with a raised border that causes it to look a bit like a paper punch has been used to make it. The sore may be on the skin in the genital area where it can be easily seen, or it can develop internally, where it may go unnoticed.

Because this lesion is not too bothersome, and if it happens to be inside a woman's vagina, she will probably not even know it is there. Syphilis, therefore, is often neglected and left untreated. When untreated, the germ will slowly migrate through the bloodstream or body tissues to any part of the body where it lies dormant. Years later, a crippling form of arthritis may develop, a serious brain infection causing permanent loss of normal mental functioning can occur, or a baby born to an untreated syphilitic mother is almost certain to have serious birth defects. The other results are too many to list. The important fact is that syphilis can be cured. It needs careful, long-term follow-up, but it is completely curable.

Herpetic VD

A fairly new venereal disease is called "herpetic VD." It is caused by one of several viruses that also cause cold sores or fever blisters about the mouth and nose. Some authorities believe it has become a problem in the reproductive tract because of the fairly widespread practice of oral sex. At any rate, it is painful and it is almost untreatable. The ulcerations it causes can be cauterized with chemicals, but this is painful and may not cure it after all. As with most infections caused by viruses, however, the body does tend to fight it and recover its health.

Vaginal Infections

There are two common vaginal infections that are not usually spread through sexual intercourse, though they may be. They are caused by microorganisms called yeast and Trichomonas. Both of these infections can be easily picked up in a bathtub or from swimming. They commonly occur after long or intensive treatment with antibiotics. They produce a vaginal discharge that causes severe itching and burning. Since the urethra and urinary bladder are very close to the vagina, there may be a bladder infection as well.

Treatment of these diseases is best recommended by your physician. He can prescribe medication to be inserted in the vagina and may order oral medication to completely cure them. Though men rarely have any symptoms of these infections, they may carry the organisms. A husband and wife can bounce this sort of infection back and forth between them without any other sexual exposure. In such cases, oral treatment is necessary for both spouses.

It is unfortunate that one needs to include negative topics in a book such as this. Teaching our children about sex ought to be positive and happy. In our Western world, however, these tragedies are reality. We do have incest, abortions, and venereal disease, and you parents need to know and understand these issues.

The happy side to such information is that, in most instances, you can prevent these problems from happening to your children. Your awareness of the possibility of such tragic episodes in their lives can make you watchful and protective. Through your information and responsibility, you may teach your children more effectively. Your positive attitude will invite them to come to you before they become involved in something that could be harmful to them. This positive life cycle can be transferred to your children as they grow so that they, too, will benefit from healthy attitudes, accurate information, and a sense of responsibility.

11
Birth Control

In light of the new medical developments in the area of birth control, we need to examine this in some depth. There are many opposing viewpoints, held by profoundly honest people, about using contraception at all. In this chapter we will learn about the more common methods of birth control and their safety and effectiveness. You must decide for yourself which to use and when and how to teach your older children about them.

Birth control is an issue that keeps coming back for resolution. When God created Adam and Eve, He told them, "Be fruitful . . . and replenish the earth . . ." (Genesis 1:28). Certainly in their day that made sense. A world empty of humans except for the two of them needed some replenishing! In today's world of indescribable poverty, hunger, and overpopulation, however, there is quite the opposite problem. We need fewer people, not more.

The Roman Catholic Church, for its own respected reasons, has devoutly maintained that medical birth control is a sin. Let me define birth control as the use of artificial means to prevent conception, and not the interruption of life after conception. Roman Catholics are permitted to use the rhythm method of birth control, but are strictly forbidden to use other means. This has created a conflict for many sincere Catholics who are forced to choose between economic practicalities and church doctrines. There is an ongoing discussion among Catholic theologians, prelates, and social scientists on this matter.

Common Methods of Birth Control

The first type of birth control we will consider is called the
"rhythm method." You will remember that ovulation takes place
about midway between a woman's menstrual periods and it is
possible to become pregnant only within a very few days after
ovulation. To abstain from sexual intercourse, then, would prevent pregnancy. The problem with this method is the erratic nature of ovulation. Sometimes it occurs earlier and sometimes later.
There is now the possibility of taking one's temperature every
morning before rising. This is called the "basal temperature" and
it is one degree higher at the time of ovulation. This knowledge
helps the user of this method to be more accurate in timing. It is
also known that during ovulation, the degree of acidity and al-
kalinity of the vaginal area changes. There are simple ways by
which a woman may test this, and again, the chance of preventing
pregnancy is increased. The rhythm method at best, however, is
not a sure one.

The Diaphragm

Another method of birth control is the use of a mechanical
barrier over the cervix or the penis. In common use today is the
diaphragm, a cuplike structure made of soft rubber and held in
shape by a firm rim. It is inserted into the vagina before each
sexual contact and left in place for six to eight hours after intercourse. It covers the cervix and prevents the entry of sperm into
the womb. It is used with a gelatinous preparation that tends to
destroy sperm as well. The diaphragm, to be effective, must be
precisely fitted by a physician. This is 96 percent effective in
preventing conception.

Prophylactics

Condoms or rubbers have been used by men for many decades.
These are also made of soft rubber and are slipped over the penis
just before sexual intercourse is completed. Not only do they
prevent pregnancy but they also protect men from most venereal

diseases. Condoms are about 99 percent effective as a birth-control measure but they are inconvenient and spoil the sponaneity of lovemaking.

Nonprescription Preparations

Various foams, gels, and vaginal suppositories as well as douches have been widely used as a form of birth control. They generally work by killing the sperm cells, washing them out, or preventing them from entering the womb. These preparations can be purchased without a doctor's prescription, are usually harmless, but are not very effective in preventing pregnancy. Often young people experiment with them, falsely thinking that they are safe from a pregnancy.

The Pill

For about three decades, birth control has been possible through hormonal intervention in the form of a pill. By understanding accurately the complex hormone cycle that begins menstruation at puberty, doctors have discovered how to safely prevent the process of ovulation. The ovaries are simply put at rest, until a couple is ready for a child. By stopping "the Pill," as it is commonly called, in a few weeks or months, the woman has reestablished her normal cycle and may become pregnant. This is almost 100 percent effective, is relatively safe, and only requires that a woman never forget her pill. According to her normal cycle, she will take a pill every day for twenty-one days. Upon stopping them, she will have a menstrual period and will again take the pill for twenty-one days. She needs to have regular medical examinations to be sure that she is not having any negative reactions.

The few side effects of the Pill need to be understood. Some women suffer mild nausea and tend to eat more to get rid of that uncomfortable sensation, causing weight gain. Most women gain a few pounds of fluid in their tissues, similar to that just before their menstrual period, and on lower doses, about midway through the month's supply of pills, they may have a little vaginal bleeding, called "breakthrough" bleeding. This means that the doctor needs to adjust the dosage. All of these problems may be solved by medical advice. The much-publicized possibility of blood clots being caused by the Pill is less than the risks of a normal pregnancy. Pills that may stop the manufacture of sperm by men are under study, but are not yet perfected or available.

It is also probable that in the next few months or years, a tiny pellet of the chemical contained in the Pill may be inserted through a tiny incision in the skin, and will slowly release the substance without a person's even having to take a pill!

There is a hormone, commonly called the "morning-after pill," that can destroy the fertilized ovum as long as three days after intercourse. It is especially useful in cases of rape or incest. This pill does not prevent conception and therefore is less desirable than the methods previously mentioned. It also causes such severe nausea and discomfort that it could not be used on a regular basis.

The IUD

The most common method for preventing the implantation of the ovum is the IUD, or intrauterine device. It is a coil of fine plastic that is inserted into the womb. Without injuring the tissues, it moves about just enough to prevent the egg from settling into that soft lining, establishing its nurturing system of blood vessels, and instead it causes the egg to be discharged from the womb. Recently, there has been concern among some medical authorities about the safety of the IUD. Women who use or are considering the use of this method should consult their doctors for more information.

Medical science has studied and perfected safe methods of birth control. By the use of these proven methods, the sexual enjoyment of a husband and wife may be greatly enhanced. The ability of today's couple to plan the size of their family may enrich the quality of life for everyone.

Family Planning

Some idealistic couples believe that God, who is Lord of all, surely is able to give them only the children He wants them to have. They feel that preventing conception takes away from their total dependence on God. While I believe God can do anything He chooses, I do not often see Him interfering with His own natural laws. In a world as overpopulated as ours, if every couple had a child every year (and that is quite possible), for some twenty years, the problems of world hunger and poverty would multiply beyond correction. Statistics show that in order to even hold the population where it is, without reducing it at all, each family needs to be limited to two children. In the Orient, there are financial motivators by the government that give tax exemptions for two children, but heavy penalties for more than two. It may be socially irresponsible, therefore, for couples to have large families.

John Kepler, scientist and astronomer, said in worship and wonder, "O, God, I am thinking Thy thoughts after Thee." Surely God has inspired scientific progress with amazing rapidity in recent decades. Very few Christians refuse to take antibiotics when they are ill, and because of medical discoveries, life expectancy has doubled in about fifty years. Health and the quality of life have been enhanced immeasurably. Careful family planning seems to belong in the category of increasing the quality of life. It seems responsible and wise to use the means God has provided to plan our families.

Teaching Teens About Contraceptives

Birth-control measures have their disadvantages as well as their advantages. Not only are they effective for married couples but also for singles and those who want to have affairs outside of marriage. The risk of unwanted pregnancies used to serve as a deterrent to such a way of life. Now that people can almost totally prevent such pregnancies or easily abort the rare one that happens, sexual promiscuity is a reality.

So far this chapter has been written for your information as parents. There is a point, however, where you need to teach your older children about contraceptives. They certainly need to know by the time they are considering marriage. But in practicality, they may need to know much sooner.

When we know that almost 50 percent of high-school girls have had sexual intercourse before graduation, we know that at least one out of every two girls needs to understand how to prevent pregnancy. The statistics for boys are even higher. Many thoughtful people are looking hard at teenage sexual practices, and the permissiveness that has allowed such premature activities. Hopefully we can educate our children so well that they will reverse the trends and decide to postpone sex until they are ready for marriage.

Until that day comes, however, you need to speak openly with your children. Encourage them to be responsible enough to avoid sex until marriage, but be aware that they may not. Temptation is present in the form of peer pressure, the media, and the values of today's liberal society. Another level of being responsible means, therefore, that you have provided your children with adequate information about birth control.

You may believe that by teaching your teenager about birth control you are, theoretically, providing him a basis for being sexually active. That will not happen if you have taught him the entire concept of this book. By showing him your own wholesome attitudes, sharing accurate information with him, and developing in him a sense of responsibility, you will finish the cycle of your own maturity. Giving him guidelines about contraception will only complete his sex education.

12
Homosexuality

Since the advent of "Gay Rights" and the resistance there has been to this movement, homosexuality has become a common household term. Teachers of kindergartners have told me that five-year-olds talk to each other about "queers" in terms that show they understand what being "queer" is. Most parents have a horror of their child's becoming homosexual, and yet they do not know what causes it or how to prevent it. Everything from genes and chromosomes to demons has been blamed for this condition, and there is actually very little that we know about it. However, there are some factors that we can define, and it is certain that some discussion of homosexuality should be included in this book.

For many years, homosexuality was listed as a sexual abnormality in the *Diagnostic and Statistical Manual* of the American Psychiatric Association. Under great pressure from various sources, however, the latest revised edition of this manual no longer lists it as such. There is still intense disagreement among qualified physicians regarding this change. Since the biological purpose of sex is reproduction, homosexuality may be considered biologically abnormal to some degree, because its purpose is never reproduction. Homosexuality is extremely rare in the animal world.

It is vitally important, at this point, to clarify that except in the area of sexual functioning, many homosexuals are fine and quite normal people. It is unfortunate that in defining the abnormality and heartache of homosexuality, many people have shown hatred for homosexual persons. Such animosity is undeserved and contradictory to the very Bible that is used to condemn them.

In order to help increase our understanding of homosexuality, let's discuss some of the theories and facts that are involved in the making of a homosexual.

Causes of Homosexuality

Negative Parental Influence

A friend of mine is chief of the Department of Child Psychiatry in a state-university medical school. In a recent lecture, he suggested that an infant's parents, especially the mother, assign to him what he called the "core gender." That is to say, by their unconscious preferences, they will treat a child, despite its anatomy and physiology, as though it were the sex they wanted it to be. According to this theory, a boy whose parents wanted a girl will be treated as a girl is treated. He will be petted and handled gently like a girl instead of tossed and roughhoused as most parents treat a boy. As he grows, he will be dressed in feminine style and will learn to talk like a girl, play, and in general, act like a girl. Even his toys will tend to be those girls are taught to play with. It is easy to see how such a boy will tend to prefer playing with girls, and at puberty, will intuitively want to date another boy. With a girl, of course, the reverse will be true. This theory is evident in many families with whom I have worked.

The family of a nine-year-old boy came to a clinic at the recommendation of his teacher. She was concerned about the child's discomfort around boys and noticed that he acted like and seemed comfortable only around girls. Since girls of nine usually believe all boys have "cooties," they ostracized him, and Terry was a lonely, miserable child.

As we investigated the family, we found a somewhat cold though conscientious mother. She was definitely in control of her family, and the boy's father, who traveled much of the time, allowed her to take charge even though he felt she overprotected

Terry. He was concerned about his son's becoming something of a "sissy."

As a preschooler, Terry was wild with delight, playing in the mounds of dirt next door, where a new house was being built. As soon as she saw him playing in it, however, his mother dragged him, screaming, into the bathtub, cleaned him, and dressed him up. In a desperate search for his mother's love and approval (having given up, apparently, on getting these from his "long distance" father), Terry had slowly but surely given up his normal boyishness and was learning to be like her. He became the little girl his mother unconsciously wanted. Fortunately, at his age this was reversible. His father spent time teaching Terry how to be a man, and in the process, the two also became friends. His mother realized how unfair her expectations were and discovered that she really could accept the masculinity of her son.

Much of my early psychiatric teaching was done by Doctors Karl and Will Menninger from the well-known Menninger Clinic. Few people in the psychiatric specialty have enjoyed the enduring and universal respect that these men so deserve. They believe that it is approximately between two and five years of age that a child develops the sense of sexuality. The qualities of maleness or femaleness, as they are defined by the parents' way of life, are learned and imitated in miniature. The early mannerisms and habits become fixed as the child grows. To have this happen in a normal fashion, a child needs to have some enjoyable time with the parent of the same sex, with the approval of the parent of the opposite sex.

Had little Terry been able to spend time with his dad exploring the new house next door, pounding nails, perhaps, or playing unhindered in the tempting piles of dirt, his problem probably never would have developed. And had his mother enjoyed his exuberance and temporary dirtiness, even his father's absence may not have played such an important part in damaging his life.

A beautiful fifteen-year-old girl came to me for psychiatric help because she was depressed and suicidal. She soon revealed that she was a lesbian and told me this story. She had been conceived and born to a young mother who was not married. Such behavior was intolerable to her family, though they tried to take care of her and the baby. The young mother continued to be irresponsible and rebellious, totally rejected her little girl, and strained her relationship with her parents. As the child grew, she resembled her mother very closely. She reminded her grandmother so much of her daughter's rebelliousness and all the pain she had brought her parents that she, too, rejected this lonely child. It was only the girl's grandfather who could love her. He took her on long walks in the park, taught her to carve sticks into little men, and told her stories at night. No one taught her to cook or sew or clean house. As she grew up, Elisa only knew how to be like her grandfather, and as she reached puberty her developing sexual desires caused her to reach out to girls, just as a normal boy would do.

When a parent teaches a young child that all people of the opposite sex are bad, stupid, or undesirable, the child will tend to believe this is true. This is especially so when that parent is powerful and threatening. And this belief is totally convincing to the child when the other parent's way of life seems to prove the first one right.

Luke was the child of such parents. He came to see me because he wanted to overcome his homosexuality. He was in his late teens and remembered, from early childhood, hearing his mother insult men in general, and his father in particular. According to her outbursts, all men were stupid, slow, and generally incompetent. Luke remembered that when his dad tried to fix a leaky faucet, a fountain sprayed the bathroom. The stopped-up drain in the basement backed up foul-smelling sewage when his father tried to clear it. Luke loved his slow-moving, patient father. But in his family, he could tell it didn't pay to be like him. So Luke watched his efficient, aggressive mother. He discovered that pleasing her kept him out of trouble and gained her approval. But pleasing Mom, as Luke saw it, meant being like her. As much as he could, Luke became like her. Later, to his own and his parents' horror, Luke had become so closely identified with her that he was a homosexual.

Many homosexuals state that they are perfectly happy in their life-style. Homosexual patients with whom I have worked, however, tell me that this is not always true. They describe lives haunted with the fear of rejection, jealousy, and endless anger. They say it is a superficial life-style, in which a person pretends to please a partner for his immediate gratification. He may even yearn for a lasting and meaningful relationship. It is common, however, to suffer repeated losses of partners as each person becomes involved in a desperate search for happiness that requires more and more effort, but gains less and less satisfaction.

The above examples are disguised from real-life experiences to protect wonderful people. In each of these and many more, the common factors in the family are these: an angry, controlling parent, and a more passive, "peace at all costs" parent; a parent who is powerful and unconsciously threatening paired with one who acts and feels afraid and incompetent. The homosexual person, growing up in such a negative atmosphere, must struggle with both fear and anger. In my experience, a major emphasis in therapy must be the healing of the hurts that came from troubled family relations.

Harmful Childhood Experience

A common experience in the lives of many homosexuals is an early encounter with an older homosexual. Matt had some of the marks of an effeminate youngster when he joined scouting. He was trying hard to be a "regular guy" and was beginning to feel pretty good when the troop went on an overnight camp-out. The scoutmaster asked him into his tent for some help, and there he forced him into a homosexual encounter. Matt was horrified and felt that he was violated, dirty, and permanently contaminated. He was too ashamed to tell anyone, and the man had threatened to hurt him if he did tell.

Matt believed that he could never again be normal. He had not been given a good sex education by his parents, and because of many tensions between them and himself, he did not feel that he could talk to them at all. There was no one he knew to whom he could turn for comfort or help. Matt's story is repeated in the life history of a great many homosexuals.

Bakwin and Bakwin, in their book *Behavior Disorders in Children,* state that almost all people could fit on a scale of one to ten as far as their sexuality is concerned. The most heterosexual would be ones and twos. The most homosexual would be nines or tens. They believe that many people ride the fence on a scale of four to six. With social permission, the influence of a friend, estrangement from parents or other supposedly trustworthy adults, and an experience such as Matt's, they may move in one direction or the other.

This information is significant in a world as changing and unsure as ours. If a child is borderline in his sexual identity, he could easily be nudged ever so insidiously into active homosexuality by a teacher, scoutmaster, or a friend who believes this to be an acceptable or even (as one alarming textbook states) a preferable way of life. One of my homosexual patients urged me to join the fight against gay rights because he believes social permissiveness is a significant factor in some homosexuals.

Absence of Role Model

Yet another influence in the causing of homosexuality is divorce. Until very recently, children of a divorce were routinely given into the custody of their mothers. The very fact of the divorce meant that the parents had anger toward each other. To a child's simple way of thinking, "If mother's anger could get rid of Dad, I'd better be careful or she'll get rid of me." This fear of a controlling, angry parent is a common factor in homosexuals. Add to such fear the loss of a male role model and the loss of the opportunity to work through the normal conflicts of growing up with both parents, and it is likely that some divorces, at least, may produce children with borderline sexual identities.

"Borderliners" are further confused by the loss of sexual role definitions in society today. At one time, sexuality could be defined by personality traits, careers, and dress, as well as by anatomy, physiology, and X-Y chromosomes. Men used to be known as aggressive, hard driving, muscular, strong, brave, and were the leaders of any group. The jobs available to women as recently as forty years ago were largely limited to teaching, nursing, secretarial work, or domestic employment. Until the 1940s, no respectable woman wore anything but dresses and the swim wear or sportswear of those days is now a laughing matter. Hairstyles were certainly not to be confused, and the only jewelry men would wear was an occasional ring.

All of that has now changed. Women have gained access to all careers and jobs and can do them well. They can swear as much, be just as aggressive, and take charge as capably as men. The manner of dressing, hairstyles, and jewelry are so similar between men and women that one must often struggle to distinguish one from the other. Many people today must ride that borderline very closely, and it is no wonder that we see an increase in homosexuality.

Facts About Homosexuals

No one really knows how many homosexual people there are in this country. A thoughtful article in *U.S. News & World Report* in April 1980, estimates there are 20 million lesbians and gay men in the United States. The article quotes Dr. John Money, from Johns Hopkins Medical School, as saying that some 13 percent of males and 7 percent of females in America are gay.

Homosexuality is certainly not a new way of life. In Old Testament times, it was practiced as early as the days of Abraham and Lot. God's condemnation of Sodom and Gomorrah, as told in Genesis 19, was clearly related to the practice of homosexuality and violence. The word *sodomy,* in fact, is named after that ancient city. In the New Testament, homosexuality is specifically condemned as sinful by Paul in his writings.

According to a report from a venereal-disease specialist in a large midwestern city, some 80 percent of all the reported cases of syphilis are found in homosexuals. The physician believes this is due to increased aggressiveness in the homosexual as compared with heterosexual partners.

An article in *Time,* March 24, 1980, describes several facets of violence in the gay world. The article quotes a number of observers and researchers who have found the sadomasochistic tendencies of homosexuals to be significantly higher than in heterosexuals. (Sadism is the urge to inflict pain in order to achieve sexual fulfillment. Masochism is the need to feel pain as part of sexual gratification.)

The currently popular movie *Cruising* depicts the extreme violence of murders and mutilation among homosexuals. John Devere, editor in chief of the gay magazine *Mandate,* is quoted in the *Time* article. He served as an extra in this movie and said he was "conscious-stricken" in the role, "not because the movie was being made, but because the violence the movie depicts is uncomfortably close to anyone who frequents the night world in any gay area." He added, "The enemy is not *Cruising;* it is not outside. The heart of darkness is within, after all. I'm saddened by that, and frightened for us all."

Every homosexual male and several of the lesbians I have counseled, agree that their lives and those of every homosexual they know are intensely unhappy. They live with fear of rejection, extreme jealousy, and anger over their plight.

Obviously, such violence is not true of many homosexuals, and on the other hand, it is true of a large number of heterosexuals. All of us are capable of violence and destructiveness if we allow anger and bitterness to grow within us.

Preventing Homosexuality

Homosexuality is one of the most difficult of all psychological conditions to cure. In fact, many psychiatrists will only attempt to help the gay person to live more comfortably with the problem. Because of this fact, it becomes of paramount importance that parents prevent the development of homosexuality in the first place. There are four issues that I believe to be essential in prevention.

Attitude

You as parents must have a good attitude toward both men and women in all phases of life. I hope you have seen how true that is in all areas of teaching your child about sex. As important as your attitudes are elsewhere, they are of utmost concern in the prevention of homosexuality.

As you review the examples above and the situations you may know, you will almost certainly find that the parents' attitudes were warped in some way. Elisa's grandmother, torn with grief over her daughter's wayward life, rejected her granddaughter. Her attitude said, "I can't stand you. You are like your mother!" And that mother, in her own selfish neglect of Elisa, showed her, "Girls are bad!" On the other hand, her grandfather's quiet gentleness invited her, without a word, to become like him—a man. How can Elisa be blamed for the results of that tragic drama?

How do you parents feel about your own sexuality and that of your spouse? If you resent being who you are or feel that everyone of the opposite sex is bad, your attitude will show. Your child is likely to agree with you and reject himself accordingly.

You may look back through your life to understand the origin of your negative feelings. Probably someone unknowingly taught you the same mistaken ideas by the way they treated you. There are many reasons you may have negative attitudes toward maleness or femaleness. You may already know where your poor attitudes originated, or you may need counsel with a pastor or a professional therapist to understand and change them, but it is essential that you do so. Once your attitudes and feelings are positive toward both sexes, you can experience warmth and acceptance of both. Then you will be able to accept your child, boy or girl, exactly as he or she is.

Teaching

As a parent, you need to take time and find opportunities to teach your child the basic facts about sexuality. Recently I asked a friend who knew many homosexuals what he believed parents could do to prevent homosexuality in their children. His reply was profound: "Help parents understand so they can teach their children that all of us have within us some feminine traits and some masculine traits. Teach the children to understand that it is normal to have some of both of these qualities so they need not feel guilty or different because of this."

This man was aware that one of the common factors in the experiences of most homosexuals is the constant disapproval of a parent. And one of the frequent focuses of that disapproval relates to the child's early masculinity or femininity. A boy who is more gentle and less aggressive may be seen by his parents as a "sissy," and in their efforts to make him "tough," they may drive him, paradoxically, to become even more effeminate. Several parents I know worried excessively because their little girls had become tomboys, preferring jeans and tree climbing to dolls and tea parties.

Even in body build and muscular development, some boys and girls may resemble the typical person of the opposite sex more than their own. By their worry or disapproval in this regard, parents may unwittingly drive their children into a sexual role reversal.

Teaching children that such interests and differences are acceptable will enable them to be comfortable with their uniqueness. With acceptance and love, each child may become his own kind of boy and her own special type of girl. You may guide them within the boundaries of their individuality to be the finest boy and girl they can be.

Example

You must find time to spend with your child, showing him or her how an adult of that sex acts. Teaching a child verbally is necessary as his mind unfolds, in order to give him understanding. But it is even more important that you show him by your example. It goes without saying that your words and your example must be consistent.

Fathers, let your little boys work and play with you. Let them see the sort of man you are—and that doesn't mean you must be perfect! It is delightful to watch my grandson push his toy lawn mower, wield his little golf clubs, and sit in his daddy's boat. Even at two years of age, Andy knows many of his father's activities and how to mimic them. His mother's noticing these and complimenting him completes a lesson in how to be (for him) a man, and that is wonderful. Between the ages of two and five this is extremely important. The patterns traced then will become almost permanently engraved as the child matures.

Mothers, you need to let your little girl help you about the house. It is inconvenient to put up with the chatter and mess of a small child, and you could do your work much faster without her presence. But later, she won't have time to be with you and won't want to help. If you can keep your priorities straight, you will know that getting the work done during these few crucial years is not so important as getting your daughter to become a happy, self-accepting woman like you. As you see her develop, you may even come to like yourself, reflected in her, better than you dreamed you could. Remember that it's not just teaching her the housework you do that is important. Your daughter can learn to keep house when she wants to. It is, rather, the feminine grace with which you move, the gentle way you talk with her, and the fun of your laughter that are composing for your child a picture of the woman she is to be. Her father needs to feel proud of both of you and let you know that.

As you teach your child verbally, you will convey much to him besides the words you say. Dr. Ross Campbell, in his excellent book *How to Really Love Your Child,* says that direct eye contact is vital to good communication. You need to take time to tell your child what is good about him, his behavior, and his achievements. You may also need to tell him what is wrong about all of these and punish him. But this can be done in a loving, constructive way that will increase his self-respect, not diminish it.

Not only does a child need the sort of time described above with the parent of the same sex but he obviously also needs time with the parent of the other sex. Andy needs time with his mother to feel her approval of his miniature manliness. And he needs the sense of her warmth and acceptance to balance the masculine aggressiveness in his developing personality. He may also learn to dust, vacuum, and cook without being effeminate. It is not what people do but how they see themselves and others, and how they feel about what they see, that determines their social sexuality.

Andy, as a very little boy, is fortunate to know already how to be a man and even has some sense of the kind of woman he will someday marry.

Protection

The fourth component in preventing homosexuality is protection. We have determined that parental attitudes are of primary importance. Information relayed by words and examples confirms those attitudes. And now your responsibility is to be alert to the dangerous influences in our world. You need to join the schools in warning your children to avoid strangers. Be sure your child knows what to do if anyone ever approaches or threatens him. Have your own plan for protection that will fit your child and your neighborhood. Should anyone, strange or well-known, suggest any sexual act or threaten your child, be sure he knows what to do and where to go for safety. Younger children, of course, ought to be within sight and hearing of a protecting adult at all times.

Tragically, however, you should be aware of relatives who are often close to a child. Sexual molestation by family members, including parents and grandparents, is an alarmingly frequent happening. Especially when this is of a homosexual type, it may have devastating effects. Usually such events are wrapped in the secrecy of fear and threats, so your child may not tell you. Don't panic and don't make hasty accusations. Simply watch your child around others. His face will rarely lie, and you will detect the signs that will tell you whether or not all is well. Either your child will act worried or frightened, or he will be comfortable and relaxed. In a careful and calm manner, ask your child if a suspected person has ever upset or worried him in any way. Let him know he can come to you with any concern, no matter what anyone else may say. If you have serious doubts, keep the child from being alone with the questionable person.

You also need to be aware of baby-sitters. There are many reliable, loving young people who develop their financial and personal responsibility through baby-sitting. But be aware of the rare one who has other motives. Such people usually have "body language" signs that will alert you. They may avoid eye contact with you. Your child may show subtle signs of fear or even some nervousness or increased activity when such a sitter arrives. Listen to your child if he resists a certain sitter. It may be that your child is spoiled and wants a sitter who is easier to manipulate into a later bedtime. But it may also be true that a certain sitter is a threat to your child's safety. You need to find out and protect your child.

If your child does have a homosexual encounter or attack, hopefully you will find out. One way to be almost certain that he will come to you is by keeping your relationship so positive and your communication system so open that he can tell you. Mark was seven when, on his way home from school, he was accosted by a man. He tried to run from him, but was taking a shortcut through an alley and could not get to a house. The man pulled Mark into a shed and raped him. As soon as he could, Mark ran sobbing to his mother, pouring out his tale of woe. His mother, having previously heard various other excuses for Mark's being late, paid no attention to him and severely punished him for lying. A child who desperately needed help and protection received even more pain and punishment instead. As you may imagine, Mark developed serious emotional problems as he grew older, and struggled with his sexual identity.

While this story is extreme, it is not rare. Mark and any child who has such a cruel experience needs a parent to take care of him physically, support and comfort him emotionally, and then explain the sickness of the one who could commit such an act. The child must know it was not his fault and that he will be all right —just as good as ever. He needs to be encouraged to talk and cry out his feelings of fear, anger, or even excitement, until he no longer has anything to say. It is often wise to have a child who has suffered sexual molestation of any kind seen by a doctor and a counselor to be sure no serious damage has been done.

Many adolescents go through a phase in their social-sexual development called a "schoolboy (or girl) crush." In this time a girl (or boy) and their best friend may become so attached to each other they are inseparable. There may be some physical affection demonstrated between them, and they may even do some exploring of each other's sexual areas. Remembering the definition of the erogenous areas of the body will help you understand that such sex play may become sexually arousing. Some teenagers mistakenly believe they are homosexuals because of such an experience. By continuing this physical intimacy, a young person may form habits of homosexuality that become hard to break.

You parents need to watch your children. Teach them how to be affectionate without becoming physically intimate. Help them to feel so emotionally secure and loved that they will not be so dependent on physical touching. And be sure they know that if they do fall into sexual intimacy with someone of the same sex, they are not doomed to a life of homosexuality. They usually will outgrow such a "crush" and develop perfectly normal relationships.

Is There a Cure?

When a young person reaches puberty and finds himself truly homosexual, prevention is no longer possible. At that time or at any time, a cure can be considered if the person honestly wants help. In my experience, it is rarely that an older practicing homosexual sincerely wants to change. Even if he does, the very nature of the causative influences creates serious barriers to getting help. Due to the dominating, frightening parent, the ability to trust and work with the therapist is very hard to develop. Since the influences on the person's self-concept began so early, it may be impossible to remember enough to understand and work through the old problems and to make new decisions. Often, unconsciously, the person has used the homosexuality as a means of getting even with a parent who is seen as cruel. And commonly there is a deep, unswerving belief that in the next homosexual partner one may find the elusive ingredient that was missing with the father or mother.

One homosexual patient had an ever-recurring dream when she slept with a woman. She would feel in the dream that her mother was holding her as a little girl, tenderly, with her arm around her, while the little girl rested her head on her mother's shoulder. She would awaken to the reality that her mother, now dead, had never and would never hold her. The longing and emptiness left by a rejecting, too-busy mother were still there, and despite the search, a homosexual relationship could never fulfill that.

Once homosexuality has been firmly established as a viable life-style, humanly speaking the chances are slim that this decision can be reversed. The best solution, as we mentioned before, is in prevention and detection of early signals from a child that his sexual identity is becoming confused. If parents are alert and responsive to their children, the problem need not arise.

What to Teach Your Child About Homosexuality

Since homosexuality is open, common, and a frequent topic in the media, parents need to explain it to their children. You may simply tell them what you have read in this chapter—put into your own words, of course. Help them to understand that in most ways a homosexual is a normal human being who is intelligent, concerned, and striving for a good life. However, as a small child he was trained and taught in a way that ended up in confusion for him about his sexuality. At first he simply did not know that he was different from other children. But later, when boys and girls were beginning to be interested in the opposite sex, he realized that he was only interested in people of the same sex.

Children need to understand that this is not an idle decision made because a homosexual wants excitement or attention. Rather it is a deep unconscious sense of "being" that this person usually abhors and intensely wishes he could change. While homosexuals are called "gay" in today's vernacular, my patients tell me they are not happy. The several homosexual patients I have treated tell me that of all their personal homosexual acquaintances and friends, they do not know a single person who is glad to be gay.

Young people, then, need to be taught to love and treat a homosexual as they do any other person. They need not be afraid of him, because his sexuality is not contagious! They need not treat him as a freak because they can't understand him. They need not discuss his differentness because it is his own private concern. But if a homosexual friend wants to discuss his sexual preference, the heterosexual young person can listen and share his own feelings and attitudes openly, kindly, and without judging the other.

It is at this point that your attitudes as parents come into focus. Many people are shocked or afraid of anything that is very different from their own experience of life. If you show abhorrence, anger, or rejection of a homosexual person, your children will probably react identically. If you try to understand the person, see his pain, and love him, your children will learn from you a sense of compassion for all the "different" people in their lives.

As a parent, being intolerant of the homosexual person may have a dangerous aspect. If you happen to have a rebellious child, he may deliberately explore a homosexual life-style simply to establish his independence from you. If he is strongly heterosexual, this will be temporary and he will leave it. But if he has some tendency toward homosexuality, he may become so involved in that way of life that he finds it hard to get out.

All of this may sound very permissive, and some of you will say it is antiscriptural. Accepting a person who is ignoring all the biblical injunctions against homosexuality surely cannot be right! Let me remind you that we, as believers in God's Word, are specifically commanded to love and not to destroy people by our judgments. It is wise to recognize and reject wrong ideas, wrong actions, wrong ways of life. Avoiding these errors (or sins) as parents and training our children to a right way of life is certainly our responsibility. But to condemn or judge individuals is God's prerogative, not ours.

There is hope for the homosexual! The core of that hope is universal and it rests on the certainty of God's love and acceptance of each person who comes to Him in honesty. There are some exciting new movements to help the homosexual who wants to leave that life-style. One of these is called Exodus. The headquarters is P.O. Box 5439, Seattle, Washington 98105.

It is widely known in psychiatry that a cure for homosexuality is one of the most difficult to achieve. Long periods of psychoanalysis have been known, however, to accomplish that. In today's Charismatic movement, many people have witnessed to deliverance from homosexuality. Some of these, however, have backslidden, and the loss of their deliverance has created serious spiritual doubts. A number of homosexuals have chosen to ignore the biblical message against that life-style and have formed their own church and community.

As a Christian psychiatrist, I firmly believe and have seen that a combination of good psychiatry, an honest commitment to Christ's Lordship, and the finding of supportive friends can enable a homosexual to become a comfortable heterosexual.

The purpose of this chapter is not to teach a cure for homosexuality. That is, at best, a long, arduous process. Often it is impossible to achieve a cure. But hopefully, you have gained insight into the factors that cause homosexuality. As parents, you can prevent its occurrence in your children. In this situation, the proverbial ounce of prevention is indeed worth the pound of cure.

Furthermore, I hope you have gained a sense of compassion for the many homosexual people in our world. Due to many social and personal influences, it is predictable that there will be increasing numbers of men and women in the gay community. Sharing God's love for them is the responsibility of the Christian community.

Epilogue

I hope that every parent who reads this will discover and develop truly positive, wholesome attitudes toward sexuality and sexual intimacy. I hope your information about sexual issues has become complete enough to allow you comfort and joy in your own marriages. Furthermore, I hope you can now discuss sexual topics with your children in an appropriate and calm fashion. I trust that your sense of responsibility about teaching your children has become so deep that you will no longer wait for someone else to do that for you.

As you have grown in these areas, I profoundly wish for you to discover the wholeness that is yours as you understand what it means to be created in the very image of God. And I pray that you will share your discoveries with the other intimate people in your life so they, too, may discover their heritage as God's created children.

I know that by the law of averages, many of you were not given right attitudes or information by your parents. Some of you may have ignored or rejected the good teaching you did receive. And you may have suffered the painful results of your rebelliousness or lack of knowledge. Even after reading all of this, it may seem so difficult to change that you feel like doing nothing.

Let me urge you not to give in to this temptation to lethargy. You don't have to learn it all at once or do it all at once. Just begin with the little steps you can take. Ask God's help and seek a friend to work with you. When you fall into old habits and break your new resolve, just get up and start again. Get your priorities in order in your marriage and with your children. Practice all of your new attitudes and encourage them in your family. Keep your intellect active and add new information to what you already have. Be careful to measure truth by the guideline of the ages: the Scriptures. And maintain a sense of responsibility. These elements, used collectively, will fill a family with joy and love for one another.

Bibliography

"A New Big Push for Homosexuals' Rights." *U.S. News & World Report,* 14 April 1980, pp. 93–95.

Bakwin, Harry, and Bakwin, Ruth M. *Behavior Disorders in Children.* Philadelphia: W.B. Saunders Co., 1960.

Brown, J.F. *Psychodynamics of Abnormal Behavior.* New York: McGraw-Hill Book Co., 1940.

Campbell, D. Ross. *How to Really Love Your Child.* Wheaton, Ill.: Victor Books, 1977.

Child Study Association of America. *What to Tell Your Child About Sex.* New York: Permabooks, 1959.

Dobson, James. *Hide or Seek.* Old Tappan, N.J.: Fleming H. Revell Co., 1974.

———. *Dare to Discipline.* Wheaton, Ill.: Tyndale House Publishers, 1970.

———. *The Strong-Willed Child.* Wheaton, Ill.: Tyndale House Publishers, 1978.

Howells, John G. *Modern Perspectives in Child Psychiatry.* New York: Brunner-Mazel, Inc., 1971.

Janss, Edmund. *How to Give Your Children Everything They Really Need.* Wheaton, Ill.: Tyndale House Publishers, 1979.

Philpott, Kent. *The Third Sex?* Plainfield, N.J.: Logos International, 1975.

Swindoll, Charles. *You and Your Child.* Nashville: Thomas Nelson, Inc., 1977.

"The Gay World's Leather Fringe." *Time* magazine, 24 March 1980, pp. 74, 75.

Young, Leontine. *Life Among the Giants.* New York: McGraw-Hill Book Co., 1966.

Sooner or later, every parent is faced with the responsibility of teaching a child the facts of life. While this is most often thought of as "The Talk," it is really a process that begins in infancy and continues through adolescence.

To teach a child good sexual attitudes, parents need a certain amount of preparation and a basic knowledge of the facts. "By understanding the physical aspects, emotional impact, intellectual influences, and spiritual essentials, you may find—in a segment at a time—the ability to teach your child all about sex."

Dr. Grace H. Ketterman systematically provides the information parents need in order to instill wholesome sexual attitudes in their children. She begins where all sex education ultimately begins—with the attitudes and values of the parents—and examines the educational process at every stage of a child's life, dealing with the common concerns and problems of each developmental level.